Lawrence Tyler, PhD

Understanding Alternative Medicine
New Health Paths in America

Pre-publication
REVIEWS,
COMMENTARIES,
EVALUATIONS . . .

"**A**s alternative medicine and medical practice become more and more fashionable in American society, it becomes advisable for us to increase our understanding of the interaction of these services. Dr. Lawrence Tyler has written a readable book based on his scholarly research. He also integrates his personal experiences as a former patient and observer during his extensive professional sojourns in Asia. This work is neither an endorsement nor a condemnation of contemporary alternative medicine. It does provide considerable insight into why and how various cultural groups in the world engage in certain medical practices. Some methodologies may seem repugnant and unscientific in Western cultures, but they continue to exist in vast regions of the globe regardless of their degrees of success."

Norman C. Greenberg, PhD
Professor Emeritus of Anthropology,
Western Michigan University,
Kalamazoo, MI

More pre-publication
REVIEWS, COMMENTARIES, EVALUATIONS . . .

"*Understanding Alternative Medicine: New Health Paths in America* offers an insightful view into several aspects of the alternative therapy movement that are often overlooked, but deserving of attention. Dr. Tyler explores the political and social context of the increased use of TCM and herbal medicines—discussing both the negative consequences to endangered plant and animal species as well as concerns about the safety and effectiveness of certain substances. He also speaks to philosophical differences between several healing traditions and explores the potential for integration. This book is an important and useful resource for the libraries of both health care providers and consumers."

Karen Horneffer, PhD
Holistic Health Care Program,
Western Michigan University,
Kalamazoo, MI

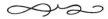

"*Understanding Alternative Medicine* is an eye-opening account of the emerging health paths in the United States and other parts of the Western world. The work surveys the new paradigm in American medical practice and consumption, identifying the growth of the 'multiple-path' approach to health care. Drawing on extensive personal experience with Asian medical traditions, Dr. Tyler outlines the traditional health strategies in India and China, contrasting them with Western philosophies of nature and medicine. Contrast turns to integration as readers explore the politics and economics of how Asian medical traditions have gained a foothold in American medicine chests and physicians' offices alongside accepted pharmaceuticals and therapies.

Special chapters are devoted to the environmental impact of the global consumer interest in 'natural' Asian medicines, with special emphasis given to the illegal overharvest of bear gallbladders and the 'poaching' of wild American ginseng in national parks. Going online, Tyler addresses the perceived efficacy and marketing of herbal alternatives on the World Wide Web, presenting revealing statistics about purity, naturalness, and standardization of many imported herbal cures.

Thoughtful discussions on the perception of 'nonspecific' factors in healing and the distance between patient and client in standard American medical practice

The Haworth Herbal Press
An Imprint of The Haworth Press, Inc.

Understanding
Alternative Medicine
New Health Paths
in America

Understanding Alternative Medicine
New Health Paths in America

Lawrence Tyler, PhD

The Haworth Herbal Press
An Imprint of The Haworth Press, Inc.
New York • London • Oxford

Published by

The Haworth Herbal Press, an imprint of The Haworth Press, Inc., 10 Alice Street, Binghamton, NY 13904-1580

Cover design by Monica L. Seifert.

Library of Congress Cataloging-in-Publication Data

Tyler, Lawrence, 1940-
    Understanding alternative medicine : new health paths in America / Lawrence Tyler.
        p.   cm.
    Includes bibliographical references and index.
    ISBN 0-7890-0741-X (hbk. : alk. paper)—ISBN 0-7890-0902-1 (pbk. : alk. paper)
    1. Alternative medicine—United States. I. Title.
R733.T94 2000
615.5'0973—dc21
                                                            99-37570
                                                               CIP

CONTENTS

ABOUT THE AUTHOR

Lawrence Tyler, PhD, is Professor of Sociology at Western Michigan University, where he teaches courses in the Asian Studies Program. From 1986 to 1987, he was a visiting professor in the Language Department at Guangxi University, Nanning, in the Guangxi Autonomous Region in China. His book, *The Blind Palmist,* is a personal account of that experience. He has been a visiting exchange professor at Nihon University in Tokyo, Japan, and has traveled throughout East Asia. Dr. Tyler is the author of several articles and has given presentations on various topics internationally.

Foreword

This book fills a long-felt need. It explains in a succinct and straightforward manner the present status of pluralistic medical care in America today.

American essayist Charles D. Warner once wrote, "Everybody talks about the weather, but nobody does anything about it." One might well apply this maxim to alternative medicine, complementary medicine, integrative medicine—whatever you choose to call it. Everyone talks about it, but very few really understand what it is. Lawrence Tyler does understand it, and his book, which explores in an analytical fashion the philosophical principles on which it is based, enables us to do the same.

Because I have spent my entire mature life dealing with botanical medicines, people are often quite surprised when I tell them that I am not an expert in the use of herbs in traditional Chinese medicine (TCM). The reason is that TCM is based on philosophical principles entirely different from those of Western medicine, and therefore requires herbs to be used in a very different manner. Lacking an understanding of the difference, most Americans view my comment with astonishment.

This book explains the important philosophical differences that differentiate native shamanism, TCM, and Indian Ayurvedic medicine, not only from conventional Western medicine but also from one another. Readers will learn how shamanism relies on a type of healing by spirits while both TCM and Ayurvedic medicine emphasize creating balance or harmony in the body, not the curing of illness.

In addition to defining the different philosophies on which various types of alternative medical treatment are based, this volume presents a unique discussion of the negative consequences of some of their practices on both the plant and animal kingdoms. A listing of a number of the ingredients used in TCM reads like a list of threatened or endangered species of flora and fauna. The premium placed on exotic natural products ranging from black bear bile to wild ginseng root threatens the very existence of these and numerous other species. In many cases, the necessary plants can be cultivated to meet market needs, but wild animals such as bears present problems that appear to be without solution, at least at present.

The book also explores the enormous recent economic growth as well as the phenomenal social acceptance of the alternative medicine industry, with particular emphasis on herbal products. The need for appropriate regulations is also discussed, with special reference to the German model. It is almost inconceivable that the United States Food and Drug Administration continues to neglect its responsibility to the health and welfare of such a large segment of the American population by refusing to evaluate properly the safety and efficacy of phytomedicines.

As noted by the author, pluralism now plays a significant role in American medicine. Further, there is every expectation that not only will it continue to do so, but that it will increase in importance in the future. It therefore behooves all of us, both professionals and laypersons, to understand the basic principles of alternative medicine. Reading this book will greatly facilitate that understanding.

Varro E. Tyler, PhD, ScD
Dean and Distinguished Professor Emeritus
Purdue University

Preface

My first encounter with traditional Chinese medicine was in Nanning, Guangxi Autonomous Region, People's Republic of China, while suffering from Bell's palsy, a bilateral paralysis of the facial muscles attributed to blockage of the seventh cranial nerve. My Chinese friends insisted that I give their medicine a try. I received both acupuncture and moxibustion, two of China's oldest therapies, used there for an amazing variety of ailments. I was taken first to an acupuncture clinic where, after insertion of the needles, the practice was to stimulate the needles with a mild electrical charge. The difficulty was in the trial and error of determining that fine line between a mild electrical current and the amount that would levitate me from the cot on which I lay. I did this three times a week for about a month. When my progress seemed marginal at best, I was advised to switch to a more traditional practitioner who positioned the needles, primarily in my face and forearm, then manually stimulated the needles by twirling them between her fingers. This practitioner also tried moxibustion as a regular part of my regimen. Moxa is essentially an herbal cigar, made of compacting and rolling a mixture of plants into a short thick stick, which is lighted to burn flamelessly but aromatically. This is then held very close to the afflicted part of the body, so that the heat, fumes, and smoke are absorbed by the patient. I was never told which of these qualities were thought to have healing properties; but since there was a distinctly hemp-like smell to the moxa used on me, I found this therapy more relaxing, though no more healing, than the previously tried electrical current.

A few years later, while living in Malaysia, I became aware that in this multicultural society there are literally thousands of bomohs or spiritual healers who draw from the pharmacopoeia and the spiritual beliefs of the Malays, Indians, and Chinese, who constitute the great majority of the population. Many are true pragmatists, who liberally draw from the folk medicines of all three traditions as well as modern medical practices.

The simple truth is that the majority of the world's population uses herbal medicines and some practice of spiritual healing in their normal medical care. Simultaneously, many simply blend available Western medicines into this multicultural approach to healing with little attempt to determine "scientifically" which works or does not work. What is of most interest to me in this study is that many Americans are beginning to do the same thing.

Perhaps due to my Asian encounters with alternative medicines, I am now, each year, increasingly aware of the growing use of alternative medicines in American society. Even small communities now tend to have a health products store and/or even an Asian products store that sells remedies to heal the sick, invigorate the tired, and soothe the stressed. If you cannot find such a shop, you can always go to Wal-Mart or Kmart, which offer many of the same remedies in prettier packaging.

The use and acceptance of alternative medicines in America is expanding exponentially. So is the misinformation. My goal in this book is to offer an alternative to misinformation and to bring some clarity to the many issues arising from the growth of alternative medicine in America.

Chapter 1

Diversity in American Medicine

The diversity of alternative medicines and medical practices in the United States is increasing in a manner that may soon alter the very definition of American medicine. The term "diversity" is primarily associated with the changing racial and ethnic composition of the population. Less attention is given to the fact that population diversity is always accompanied by a diversity of the attitudes and behaviors about basic social institutions. This diversity of attitude and behavior is now clearly evident with regard to American health care institutions and practices.

Recent population diversity has made such change inevitable as Americans of non-European origin bring their own medical pharmacopoeia and healing customs with them. The increase in the Asian-American population, especially, has been accompanied by the growing availability, awareness, and use of traditional Asian medicines, primarily Chinese-based medicine and its three traditional practices of herbalism, acupuncture, and moxibustion.

The 1990 census indicated more than 6.9 million Americans identified with the Asian-American category. The 1990 census also showed the median income for Asian-American households ($36,101) to be greater than that of white households ($30,406). Market analysts estimate that these households are a $120 billion consumer market. Asians are now one of the fastest growing groups in of the national population and are projected to represent more than 5 percent of the U.S. population by 2010. The greater part of the consumer behavior of these households is identical to that of other American households: buying Nike sportswear and stopping at McDonald's while on the way to the mall in the minivan. Yet they also represent a significant part of the less mainstream market that is fueling the growth in herbal/alternative and traditional Chinese medicines.

However, this boom of interest in Asian and other alternative medical practices is not by any means limited to Asian Americans. On the contrary, its use and acceptance among non-Asian Americans is the major source of alternative medicine growth. This is happening for at least two reasons: (1) established Western medicine is perceived by many users to have become highly impersonal, bureaucratic, and expensive; and (2) as many Americans have become preoccupied with higher levels of health and fitness, they seek the "magic bullets" and miracle cures that Western science cannot offer. Herbal medicines and alternative therapies are increasingly available options in a consumer culture geared to affluent health buffs. If blue-green algae and antioxidants are not producing the fitness level that your lifestyle requires, you can now sign up for a "Healing Practices Tour" in Nepal, or a "Chinese Herbal Medicines Tour" of Chinese hospitals, herbal gardens, and medicinal hot springs, or the "Ancient Medicines in Modern Times Tour" of India (Hainer, 1998, 5D).

The term "alternative medicine" in America today encompasses an amazing range of therapies and philosophies, literally from A (Ayurvedic medicine) to Z (Zen meditation). Other than an uneasy relationship with the American Medical Association, these often have little in common except for the tendency of their users to describe them as ways and means to a more natural health and healing.

Every society assigns positive value to nature. From the American colonial experience to the present, American writers such as Longfellow, Fenimore Cooper, Thoreau, Twain, and Hemingway have given expression to the enduring American attitude that there is a healing, redemptive power and purity associated with nature and those who live in proximity to it. As our lives become more detached from nature, it becomes easier, perhaps even emotionally necessary, to romanticize all things natural. Some historians and literary critics trace this attitude back to Rousseau and the Enlightenment philosophers who theorized about a precivilized, natural humanity "born free" of the constraints and duplicity of civilization and the social order.

If natural things are idealized in contemporary American popular culture, then herbal medicines and natural therapies, literally rooted in nature, seem by default to be unmitigated blessings. For the patients and users who have come to the pantheon of alternative medicine via this path of a romanticized nature, no teaching, preaching, or evidence to the contrary will be sufficient. But for most users and potential users of alternative medicine, there is always value in informed discourse. This book hopes to serve that purpose.

The focus of my study is to discuss this trend of the increasing use of alternative medicines in the United States (including a summary of the underlying philosophies that have guided traditional Chinese medicine and Ayurvedic medicine for centuries) and to examine two of its major consequences:

1. The environmental impact on endangered species (plant and animal) used as ingredients in traditional and herbal medicines
2. The economic growth and social acceptance of the alternative health industry

One of the first difficulties of studying the field of alternative medicine is the term itself. Especially in the United States, this term is so inclusive that it risks becoming meaningless. Some of these practices, such as traditional Chinese medicine and Ayurvedic medicine, are so ancient that, in chronological terms, modern Western medicine has developed as an alternative to them and their historical European equivalents.

In a sense, the label "alternative medicine" defines its practices in terms of what they are not. They are not conventionally accepted therapies sanctioned by the AMA. The term has been popularized both by those who think of the phrase "alternative to conventional medicine" as a compliment and by those who use it as a pejorative.

The words "complementary" and "integrative" are preferred by some, but neither appropriately applies to the great range of medicines subsumed in this category. If the Washington bureaucracy has its way, complementary will be added to alternative (as in the Center for Complementary and Alternative Medicine), in the government tradition of equating wordiness with clarity. The term complementary refers to approved drug therapies that have plant constituents as their base and to therapies such as acupuncture, in situations where they have been deemed acceptable for use along with conventional treatment.

In trying to identify the ideas that unify or are common among all the varieties of medicine labeled as alternative, the following points generally apply: (1) either explicitly or implicitly, alternative medicines assume a physical-spiritual-psychological connection by which body and mind are reciprocally influential and capable of promoting self-healing; (2) nearly all alternative medicines stress a preference for "natural" therapies and herbs along with or instead of medical technologies and drugs; and (3) all stress the importance of diet and nutrition, based on herbs and whole foods, to good health. If these three points leave out some alternative medicines, such an omission only further illustrates the difficulty of a complete definition.

Another possibility would be to use subcategories such as these:

1. Alternative oral medicines—herbals, homeopathic prescriptions, dietary supplements, etc.
2. Alternative physical therapies—acupuncture, chiropractic, massage, yoga, etc.

3. Alternative emotional/spiritual therapies—hypnosis, directed healing, spiritism, etc.

Here, of course, the difficulty is that most alternative practitioners use various combinations of these categories and are committed to holistic theories which transcend the categories. Acupuncturists, for example, are firmly committed to the theory of Qi (which is explained in Chapter 2) as the basis of acupuncture's effectiveness. Ayurvedic practitioners normally recommend all three of these subcategories.

Another possible approach would be to use the terms holistic and analytic, respectively, to differentiate between the approach to the whole person's mental/spiritual/physical health and healing associated with "alternatives," and the focus upon single disease/ailment and search for single causation and cure associated with modern conventional medicine.

The obvious problems inherent in each of these suggestions demonstrates why the term alternative medicine remains in customary usage. As vague as it is, it is at least a convenient shorthand label with wide usage. So, in the face of these limitations, this study will stick with the term alternative medicine.

Chapter 2

Philosophical Differences

Ayurvedic philosophy recounts that the god Indra knew the principles of healing even before illness came into the world of humankind. Since Indra revealed these principles to humans, the basis of health and well-being has been available here in the world for all those who have eyes to see it and ears to hear it. Thus, for the Ayurvedic physician, healing is a matter of preparing or sensitizing the patient to the path of health as well as the preparation and dispensing of herbal medicines. Ayurvedic practitioners may now include allopathic medicines and drugs along with their traditional cures, but what distinguishes this medical tradition is the attitude that, whatever the prescribed treatment, healing must be spiritual as well as physical.

Modern, scientifically based, AMA-endorsed, allopathic medicine has intentionally stripped itself of such spiritual content to drive out the quackery and charlatanism that is so easily concealed in spiritually based medicine. This rational base of allopathic medicine has led to glorious achievements in surgery, technology, drug therapy, and the scientific knowledge of physical illness. However, it has also left modern medicine with the image of an uncaring, impersonal, industrial process that often cannot effectively address the nonmaterial dimensions of sickness.

It was not always so. The emblem of modern medicine is the caduceus; the staff carried by Mercury as the messenger of the gods. Even though modern physicians are trained to think analytically and scientifically, the profession still uses a symbol which implies that healing knowledge is spiritually rooted and transmitted from the gods.

SHAMANISM

The uniquely human characteristic is the ability to create and mentally fixate on abstractions, ideas for which there are no physical referents or bases in the material world. The spiritual or sacred is one of these uniquely human abstractions found universally in our cultures. Human cultures everywhere always point beyond the physical, natural realm to something supranatural and worthy of reverence; to a higher being, ultimately mysterious, that can only be apprehended through belief, not through rational comprehension.

Something so powerful as a spirit realm requires attention and communication. Thus, in every culture's history there are individuals blessed or cursed with the abilities to communicate with the spiritual. These are shamans who claim to be, and are deemed to be, capable of communicating with the spiritual realm. Shamanism is the most ancient healing tradition.

Shamanism is part of the prehistory, history, and in some cases, the current affairs, of various cultural traditions throughout the world. Conjuring, summoning, blessing, and healing, shamans are the intermediaries between humankind and the realms beyond human control or comprehension.

The shamanistic world is itself alive and sensitive to human existence. It is a world that can be responsive to human needs, if only humans are able to communicate with it. The early Greek conceptualization of the primordial earth goddess Gaia is one version of this sort of animistic worldview. Gaia lingers within modern society through our casual or joking references to "mother earth." However, a few contemporary philosophers of science, such as James Lovelock (1988) and Rupert Sheldrake (1994), are not joking at all in proposing a modern Gaia hypothesis, in which a scientific model of the earth as a self-governing organism is presented as an alternative to the mechanistic model currently prevailing in most scientific study. Virtually all prescientific conceptualizations of the world include this sort of organismic analogy in which nature is seen as a living creature having similarities to familiar life forms.

From the shamanistic perspective, such an animate nature, properly summoned and comprehended, can respond to human needs with both physical and spiritual support. At the physical level, the animate world can respond with the practical knowledge of sustenance—food, shelter, herbal healing—for those who will study it. At the spiritual level, the animate world can offer the esoteric or secret knowledge of transcendence—visions, enlightenment, ecstasy—to those sensitive enough to comprehend.

Herbalist philosophies, whether Chinese, Ayurvedic, or European, all have origins in this animistic view of nature. Even today, many herbal practitioners do not want to abandon this spiritualist base in exchange for the laboratory science of a rational phytotherapy.

It is a long way from shamanism to scientific allopathic medicine. Modern Western medicine is a result of the historical separation of science and religion, or the secular and sacred, that distinguishes Western civilization from its Asian, African, and Native American counterparts. Modern Western medicine focuses upon the physical, material world and the expansion of practical, applied knowledge of that realm, while leaving esoteric and spiritual matters to theologians. The medicine of Western culture is necessarily as secularized as Western culture itself.

Shamanism, despite signs of revivalism in New Age and earth-based spiritualities, has lost its power over most contemporary lives. Yet it is counterproductive to simply rail against its appeal in many non-Western traditions and in the subcultures of a modern era that offers very limited spiritual comforts to its citizens.

This is the crux of a philosophical bifurcation that separates allopathic, AMA-sanctioned medicine from the great range of medical practices which now, for lack of a better term, are called alternative medicine. These so-called alternative models have roots in non-Western cultures and in the history of Western culture, as well as the fringes and subcultures of contemporary society. There is still a strong attraction for many people, including the well-educated and worldly, in the metaphors and symbolism of a living, animate world that can be responsive to our medical needs, both of the body and of the soul.

Stated simply, many people seem to want a health care system in which they can take faith as well as take pills, regardless of how efficacious the pills are. When forced to choose, some will even choose a health care system that they must take purely on faith rather than a system that offers only pills.

TRADITIONAL CHINESE MEDICINE

In Asia, since the steady influx of Western culture, most countries have practiced a mixture of Western and indigenous traditional medicines. This "medical pluralism" in which Western medicine and Asian health/healing practices are used simultaneously by patients has been the norm for decades. But for centuries, one of the most pervasive and influential medical systems has been traditional Chinese medicine (TCM).

The *Yellow Emperor's Canon of Medicine* or "Huangdi Neijing" is said to have been compiled during the Han dynasty. It is the first consolidation of all the potions, treatments, and methods of diagnosis of TCM into one text. It comprises a medical paradigm and philosophy based in the Chinese metaphysical concepts of yin and yang, the five basic elements of the physical world, the six channels or meridians of the body's energy, and the eight principal syndromes of diagnosis (Bertschinger, 1997, p. 673).

It is useful to keep in mind that centuries of Chinese medical practice preceded the compilation of the *Yellow Emperor's Canon.* In those pre-Canon times, there was no uniform theory of Chinese medicine. Instead, the rival influences of Confucianist theory, Taoist theory, Buddhist theory, regional differences, and competing lineages of medical families jealously guarding their professional secrets all contributed to a splendid medical disarray.

The *Yellow Emperor's Canon* was the largely successful attempt of the dynastic government to impose some order over conflicting schools of medicine, especially the Confucianist-Taoist disagreements. Rather than favoring one theory at the expense of the other, "bridges were built to link the two schools of thought, and, . . . during the Han dynasty, a union occurred that made the . . . doctrines appear as constituents of one system of thought" (Unschuld, 1988, p. 184).

All of Chinese history shows a preference for order (virtually any order, no matter how dogmatic) over chaos. TCM is no exception to this rule. Today elements of TCM philosophy sound, to the Western ear, inconsistent and/or illogical. However, from the perspective of Chinese culture, it is fully acceptable for seemingly contradictory paradigms to be "utilized as suitable tools by one and the same individual, and possibly, by society in general, for coping with different aspects of daily life and of a perceived reality" (Unschuld, 1988, p. 184). Modern Westerners who live their daily lives as both religious believers and scientific practitioners make a similar sort of intellectual accommodation.

However, this does mean that beneath the seemingly uniform framework of TCM (as outlined in the following pages), there is a quagmire of variation in actual practice. Furthermore, the matter of how to intellectually integrate TCM and Western medicine is a Western concern far more than a Chinese concern. The Chinese prefer to ignore the contradictions and avail themselves of the benefits of what works and what is politically acceptable.

To a large degree, the principal ideas of the *Yellow Emperor's Canon* are still considered relevant to medical treatment by the followers of TCM. Modern or Western medical treatments and drugs have just been added to the canon, rather than being seen as either a replacement or repudiation of it.

At various times in the modern era, Chinese political authorities have tried to undermine the practice of TCM, but with little success. In 1929, General Chiang Kai-shek attempted to ban TCM altogether (perhaps in deference to the Western medical training of Kuomintang party founder Dr. Sun Yat-sen). However, like most KMT edicts of that time, it showed no understanding of the realities of life in the Chinese countryside and was generally ignored. Chairman Mao Tse-tung, more in tune with the will of the Chinese people, during his own rule dictated that a combination of TCM and Western medicine was the best path. That mix of Taoist and Maoist Chinese medicine remains the prevailing view in China today. Though the philosophies of the two traditions differ radically, no effort has been made to modify TCM theory as Western methods are incorporated. Western method and medicines are simply added in, while any contradiction of theory or philosophy is ignored.

First, it is useful to understand that TCM does not claim to "cure illness" or to "kill bacteria and viruses." Instead, its stated purpose is the maintenance of well-being, or balance and harmony, in life. One of the main differences between TCM and Western medicine is that TCM does not aim to treat an illness, but rather to treat the person by restoring harmony or balance to the person's being. All conditions considered "illness" by Western medicine are perceived as harmonic imbalances by TCM.

In an affluent consumer society, this focus on harmonic balance has a result in which relatively healthy people continually use TCM, either in search of perfect fitness or to prevent illness. If sick, you use TCM to get well; if well, you use it to maintain harmonic balance and to gain in fitness. For the herbal supplements industry, this has the fortuitous effect of expanding the consumer market to include the healthy as well as the sick.

Qi

The focus on balance and harmony has its origins in the ancient Chinese perception that all Qi (energy) in the universe works on the principle of the complementary opposites of yin and yang. The source of all change and movement in the physical world is posited in the never fully achieved tendency toward equilibrium between things predominantly yin and things predominantly yang. Good health is a matter of relative balance and harmony between yin and yang tendencies within the being. Bad health is a matter of relative imbalance between yin and yang tendencies within the being. Qi is the energy that animates a person. It is ingested by breathing, eating, and drinking. Thus, bad breathing and bad diet can affect well-being.

Jing

The inherited (or in Western terms, genetically transmitted) part of health is "Jing." Jing is inherited from parents at conception. If parents are unhealthy at that time, so will be the child. Jing is finite; it cannot be increased. Aging is the diminishing of Jing and death is its depletion. Good diet and healthy practices can maximize Jing and the life span of the individual. Some Buddhist writings suggested that celibacy is a means for males to protect Jing.

Shen

The term "Shen" in Mandarin can mean spirits, ghosts, soul, or magic, but in TCM is usually interpreted as consciousness. It is the mental ability, memory, and cognition of the person and can be observed through the eyes. Shen can be replenished by sleep and rest.

The healing or therapeutic goals of TCM can be summarized as the following: to maintain or reestablish the yin-yang balance of Qi, to gain maximum use of the finite Jing, and to replenish Shen.

The Five Elements

In the West, the ancient philosophers and alchemists defined the basic elements of life as earth, air, fire, and water. The traditional Chinese cosmology identified five such elements: wood, metal, fire, water, and earth The universal Qi is believed to manifest in these five elements. All organs, tissues, functions, and systems of the body are associated primarily with one element or another. Similarly, in a logical though not necessarily edifying manner, each element is also linked with a primary imbalance, season, emotion, and color:

Element	Organs	Imbalance	Season	Emotion	Color
wood	liver, gallbladder, eyes	sourness, wind	spring	anger	green
metal	lungs, large intestine, nose, hair	pungent, dry	autumn	sorrow	white
fire	heart, small intestine, tongue	bitter, hot	summer	joy	red
water	kidney, urinary bladder, ear, bone	salty, cold	winter	anxiety	black
earth	spleen, stomach, mouth, flesh	sweet, damp	long-summer*	ratiocina-tion	yellow

Source: Cai, 1997, 685-686.

* The term long-summer refers to times when hot and humid weather lingers into what would ordinarily be the early days of autumn. Also, to some degree, this is a contrivance so that there can be five seasons to correspond to the paradigm of five elements.

The dynamic of balance and imbalance occurs in a definite pattern of interaction of the five elements:

- Wood can be unbalanced by metal.
- Metal can be unbalanced by fire.
- Fire can be unbalanced by water.
- Water can unbalanced by earth.
- Earth can be unbalanced by wood.

The Five Climatic Factors

There are also five climatic factors, which are the cyclic phases of the five elements during the seasons. TCM philosophy conceptualizes five seasons. This may be primarily to correspond to the five elements; or it may be because the number four is generally thought by Chinese to be unlucky. In either case, they interact in the following pattern:

Element	Season	Climatic Factor	Organ Affected
wood	spring	wind	liver
fire	summer	heat	heart
earth	long/late Summer	dampness	spleen
metal	fall	dryness	lungs
water	winter	coldness	kidney

The Eight Patterns of Imbalance

The traditional Chinese physician will attempt to diagnose the patient by assessing the eight patterns of imbalance:

- 1 + 2, interior or exterior. These refer to the location of primary ailments, whether they are associated with internal organs or with body surface and epidermis.
- 3 + 4, cold or hot. These are the symptoms of fever or chills; pallid or flushed complexion, etc.

- 5 + 6, empty or full. These are body responses such as exhaustion, fainting, and loss of consciousness, or frenzy and hyperactivity.
- 7 + 8, dryness or moisture. Does the patient complain of dehydration and thirst, or bloat and diarrhea?

The physician's goal in diagnosis will be to discern the patterns of imbalance (not disease or illness in the Western sense) and to reestablish equilibrium/harmony, ideally on all eight conditions but mainly on the pattern considered in the physician's judgment to be the most imbalanced.

The Four Diagnostic Methods

To do so, the physician will utilize four diagnostic methods:

1. *Visual observation.* The physician may carefully observe the spirit, complexion, and posture of the patient; also the texture and coating of the tongue, eyes, ears, and excreta.
2. *Sensory monitoring.* This involves listening to the patient's voice and respiration, and smelling body odor.
3. *Questioning.* This involves asking the patient about symptoms, personal habits, and family history.
4. *Palpation.* The physician will feel the pulses and body of the patient.

When a diagnosis is determined, the physician will then invariably prescribe one, or a combination, of the three classic treatments of TCM:

1. *Acupuncture/acupressure.* The stimulation by needle or pressure of "blocked" Qi at the various intersections of the energy channels of the body as hypothesized in TCM.
2. *Moxibustion.* Involves the burning of plant/herbal materials in close proximity to the affected energy points of the body.

Through absorption of either the heat or fumes, the body is thought to benefit.

3. *Herbal medicines.* Almost always prescribed in combinations; they are not prepared by standardized formula (one strength fits all) but according to the judgment of the herbalist and the need of the patient. (Ironically, in this sense, all mass-produced herbal medicines violate a basic premise of TCM.)

In TCM, when a plant or animal part is prepared as a medicine, it is always in conjunction with other ingredients. The "active" ingredient, whether ginseng, bear bile, or something else, is always consumed or ingested as part of a potion of complementary ingredients. (In traditional jargon, the active ingredient is referred to as "king" or "ruler"; the supporting ingredients as "minister," "aides," and "messenger.") Usually the active ingredient, especially any rare ingredient such as bear bile or tiger bone, is present in very small amounts to be consumed over long periods to slowly reestablish yin-yang harmony.

The interpretation of herbal ingredients as analogous to participants in a social relationship probably has its source in the ancient Chinese tendency to view the body and its organs as a microcosm of the social order. The traditional Chinese view of the social order is hierarchical; Confucian theory, especially, emphasizes class differences and inequities. In the Confucian view, social harmony is enhanced by a recognition and acceptance of unequal but necessary social roles and statuses. Thus, by analogy, herbs also are participants in a hierarchy of inequity based in their respective curative functions and purposes.

The specific details of the herbal hierarchy, however, have been especially vulnerable to various political interpretations. Very early sources refer to the ruler ingredient as dedicated to the maintenance of harmony within the organism. The ruler was also characterized as contributing to longevity. Since wisdom may be acquired through a long life, both Confucian and Taoist philosophies valued old age. Taoist alchemists sought to attain immortality through arcane potions that often included sprinklings of gold dust. (Today this is reemerging, as sumptuous meals sprinkled with gold dust are again available to the nouveau riche capitalists of China in Beijing and Shanghai restaurants.)

In the post-1949 People's Republic of China, however, the herbal relationships began to be expressed in more socialist terms in which the power of the ruler is only effective when ameliorated and filtered through the minister, aides, and messenger. Thus, over the years, TCM has been complicated by the shifting fates of a politicized pharmacology:

> Not surprisingly, pharmaceutical thinking based on Confucian values sees so-called "ruler" (chun) drugs as instrumental in the elimination of illness, assisted by "minister" (ch'en), "aides" (tso) and "messenger" (shih) drugs. Taoist oriented pharmaceutical literature used an identical terminology to express an opposite image of an ideal society: here it is the task of the lower ranks of "aides" and "messengers," and, to a limited degree only, of "ministers," to actually cure illness, that is solve crisis, while the ruler has but the function of guaranteeing harmony by doing as little as possible. It should be noted that during the Cultural Revolution in the 1970s, publications appeared in the People's Republic of China adapting the former ruler-minister-aides-messenger terminology in Chinese pharmaceutics to the social ideology dominating then. The four hierarchical levels were redefined as chu (as in chu-hsi, "chairman"), fu ("helper"), tso ("aide"), and shih ("messenger"). (Unschuld, 1988, p. 180)

This combination of many ingredients (ruler, minister, aides, and messenger) is one of the reasons that it is difficult for Western scientific testing to isolate and prove or disprove the therapeutic value of such herbal medicines. In fact, under laboratory analysis many such potions prove to have fraudulent ingredients instead of the purported contents. Such scientific proof or disproof, however, is of little concern to TCM users, who are content to accept anecdotal examples as proof of herbal efficacy.

In the United States, the Dietary Supplement Health and Education Act of 1994 was intended to clarify such matters. However, it is also a product of political compromise, not between Taoism and Confucianism but between the FDA and the dietary supplements lobby. Consequently, most herbal products are categorized as dietary supplements or food products. As such they can be sold and advertised with vague statements that the product has nutritionally desirable results or is supportive of well-being, and so on. However, all such statements must be followed up by the disclaimer that "this statement has not been evaluated by the Food and Drug Administration. This product is not intended to diagnose, treat, cure, or prevent any disease."

The Chinese Diet

Two equally long-standing practices characterize the Chinese attitude toward food. First, the Chinese eat virtually anything. Second, they attribute many medicinal consequences to this omnivorous diet.

The saying throughout Asia is that the Chinese "eat any creature that has its back to the sun." (Like most folk aphorisms, while not precisely accurate, its meaning is clear.) In other words, the encyclopedic and sophisticated cuisine of China stops just short of cannibalism. Chinese culture prides itself on an elaborate culinary tradition in which bears, monkeys, reptiles, and any creature of the sea, air, or land that attracts the attention of a Chinese chef can be turned into a great delicacy. The Confucian ethic places humans at the top of a long and varied food chain. It is difficult to think of an animal or plant that is prohibited from consumption by Chinese for moral or ethical reasons. Buddhism, a philosophy of Indian origin that many practitioners interpret as prescribing vegetarianism, is the only ethical or moral constraint on the Chinese appetite. One of the traditional expressions of wealth in China is the consumption of rare creatures and precious materials. The nouveau riche of the new economy in the People's Republic are again indulging themselves (illegally but openly) in bear paws, live monkey brains, tiger meat, and the sprinkling of gold dust over dishes of food. "Conspicuous consumption" in the most literal sense is a long-standing Chinese culinary tradition.

Recently in San Francisco, this led the city government to establish the Live Animals for Food Subcommittee to study the issue of Chinatown markets stocking various live animals for human consumption. So far this has not proven to be an issue that a subcommittee can effectively resolve to the satisfaction of either the animal rights advocates or the defenders of Chinese cuisine (Golden, 1996, p. 5A).

Concomitant with these eating customs is the equally old and powerful recognition of a close association between eating and health. The Chinese dislike of dairy and cheese products is undoubtedly rooted in mainland China's absence of refrigeration and the inability to safely store such foods. One of Mao Tsetung's first edicts to the Communist Party and to China was a prohibition against the drinking of unboiled and/or cooled water. To this day, all water in mainland China is recognized as unsafe for consumption if not boiled and still warm to the touch. Some food products, such as soybean, were first cultivated for medicinal use. Tea leaves are still viewed as either a beverage or a medicinal potion depending on their preparation. Nearly all Chinese foods are classified as "heating" or "cooling," and thus useful in balancing yin and yang, although the average Chinese is quite individualistic in assessing the heating or cooling powers of various foods.

Perhaps the most positive feature of TCM is that it has firmly established in the minds of its followers a definite and enduring association between diet and health, however idiosyncratically that association is defined.

In the grossest sense, the TCM market is the largest potential market in the world. It includes the 1.2 billion people of mainland China (20 percent of the world population), 80 to 90 million Taiwanese and overseas Chinese, and most of the 7 million Asian Americans, as well as the many converts in the general U.S. population.

AYURVEDIC MEDICINE

Ayurvedic herbalists, part of a tradition in every way as ancient as TCM, also use the metaphor of rulers and ministers in discussing herbal medicines. Again, by thinking of the body as a microcosm of society, one may treat disease at the ministerial level, with an herb for each ailment, or one may treat at the sovereign level with an herbal potion that would defeat "all ministries of illness" (Burghart, 1988, p. 293).

The Ayurvedic view is that modern allopathic medicine treats only at the ministerial level, with a drug for each disease, while Ayurvedic medicine may do this as well but is superior because it can also offer sovereign cures for the root cause of all ministerial-level ailments. It is holistic, with the view that an ailment of any part of a person is interrelated to the other parts and their functioning. Therefore the Ayurvedic practitioner may prescribe proper behavior and religious ritual along with medicines and good diet. Its medical theory is as complex and articulated as Hindu cosmology but comes down to a view of the importance of integration and balance in the process of living. Since each person is a microcosm of the universe, every action of the individual has consequences in the macrocosm and in the intricate web of living things. Awareness of this relationship to the universe is the key to individual health and well-being.

In Ayurvedic tradition, the original medical knowledge was conveyed by the god Indra, out of compassion for humankind. Since all medicine has its roots in this divine source, many Ayurvedic practitioners do not hesitate to incorporate aspects of modern allopathy. After all, from this perspective, modern, Western physicians are simply heirs of the Ayurvedic tradition who have forgotten the origin of their knowledge. Burghart (1988) quotes one Ayurvedic practitioner as saying of modern doctors, "The more forgetful they are, . . . the more wondrous appear their discoveries" (p. 297).

Three Doshas

Ayurvedic theory is most at odds with modern medicine in its conceptualization of the three doshas or types of body structure and metabolism. The vata, pita, and kapha doshas are descriptively detailed in Ayurvedic treatment. Each refers to a body build, metabolic rate, and emotional and behavioral disposition. The premise is that each person has a constitution that is dominated by one of the doshas, but also includes traits of the other two doshas. Only skilled practitioners are capable of making this determination. The subtleties of the doshas and subsequent diagnosis are lost on the casual observer of Ayurveda; only those who have made the study of such concepts their life's work are qualified to perceive them. Any attempt to summarize the doshas sounds foolishly simple. In practice, no system based in Hindu cosmology is simple.

What is more translatable to Western thought and pertinent to understanding is the Ayurvedic view that health is a harmony easily unbalanced by physical, psychological, and social influences upon a person. Disease can come from three influences—external, internal, and karmic. External sources of illness include the environment, bodily injury, and spirit possession. Internal illnesses manifest from bad diet, overwork, indulgence, and sexual misconduct. Karma is often explained in shorthand as the idea that all of our actions have consequences. However, karmic disease is not limited to the concept of a reaction to every action. Not only can we accrue bad karma from our own bad action, but from indiscretions in a past life, and even from the etheric realm where the self (and all other selves) resides between earthly cycles. A concept so pervasive, yet ethereal, as karma could easily become the crutch of lazy diagnosticians, but in practice should never be invoked except when all other diagnostic possibilities are eliminated. Overused karmic diagnosis could easily make the entire medical enterprise meaningless. Such undermining and denying of the significance of individual human effort would lead to a patient's sense of futility, and in itself would be a negative karmic act (Desai, 1997, p. 671).

Diagnosis

Once a practitioner has identified the dosha of the patient, diagnosis can proceed. The practitioner will base the diagnosis on the following activities:

1. Physical observation—especially of the tongue, eyes, and nails.
2. Questioning—about both family and personal history.
3. Palpation—feeling the body.
4. Examining urine—for color and odor.
5. Listening—to heart, lungs, and intestines.
6. Taking pulses—Ayurvedic medicine detects several pulses in the wrist.

Three Treatments

The three classic treatments are as follows:

1. *Cleansing/detoxifying* (shodan). This may include purging, elimination through the bowels, blood cleansing by bleed-

ing, the use of blood-thinning herbs, and nasal cleaning. All of these are efforts to remove toxins from the body.
2. *Palliation* (shaman). These techniques include herbs, fasting, chanting, yoga, meditation, and sunning. All are efforts to reestablish the proper balance of the dominant dosha and the two subordinate doshas within the person's constitution.
3. *Rejuvenation* (rasayana). These involve the use of tonics to revitalize the metabolism. Such medicines may be liquids, pills, powders, or jellies.

In both the shaman and rasayana forms of treatment, herbs are an integral part of a physical-spiritual therapy. According to tradition, herbal medicines are not as effective when taken outside this regimen. However, as stated earlier, some modern practitioners (Deepak Chopra is the most celebrated) have combined the spirit of these traditions with essentially modern practice to create what they consider to be the best of both healing worlds.

HERBS AND THE ICE MAN

One clear observation from this discussion is that there are several herbal traditions. Herbology is firmly rooted in TCM, Ayurvedic, and Western medicines, not to mention Native American and Afro-Caribbean healing traditions. The argument can be made that there is more hard evidence for the longevity of herbal medicine than for any other medical technique.

In 1991, in the Alps of northern Italy, a mummified body was discovered in an ice field. Testing dated the remains back to the early Copper Age, more than 5,000 years ago. Among his well-preserved possessions were two walnut-sized wads strung on a leather thong. Through laboratory analysis, these have been identified as pieces of birch fungus, *Piptoporus betulinus,* which contains oils that are toxic to certain parasitic bacteria. Scientists also know that the man had whipworm, *Trichuris trichiura.* In a

1998 *Lancet* article, Dr. Luigi Capasso writes, "The discovery of the fungus suggests that the Ice Man was aware of his intestinal parasites and fought them with measured doses of *Piptoporus betulinus*" (Capasso, 1998, p. 1864).

"Measured doses" may be reading too much into the findings, but these discoveries do strongly suggest an awareness of the medicinal powers of herbs dating back 5,000 years. This does not rule out an equally strong reliance on spiritual medicine and shamanistic charms. Very likely the herbal and shamanistic healing of 5,000 years past would have been a unified process reflecting an animistic worldview. So our Ice Man would not have been rationally weighing milligrams as so much as invoking the world of nature as he understood it.

Chapter 3

TCM Use and Endangered Species

A close relationship exists between the ingredients of many traditional Chinese medical remedies and the flora and fauna currently listed as endangered species. Asiatic black bear, leopard, musk deer, pangolin, rhinoceros, and tiger—is this a list of "active ingredients" in countless Chinese traditional medicines or is it a short list of threatened/endangered species? It is both. Ginseng, Chinese magnolia, eucommia, astragalus, *Achyranthes bidentata* —this is a list of flora commonly used in traditional Chinese medicines, and also a group of plant species now listed as vulnerable, threatened, or endangered. Although the importation to the United States of medicines that include ingredients from endangered species is illegal, trafficking in such remedies continues and is estimated to be worth hundreds of millions of dollars per year.

Gaski and Johnson (1994, p. 5) report that the "current world value for medicinal herbs has an estimated annual value of U.S. $10 billion." Patented or mass-produced Asian medicines are an important part of this but, because so many are illegal in the United States, there are no official or accurate statistics on their trade value. From 1984 through 1992, the U.S. Fish and Wildlife Service reported intercepting 1.8 million medicinal items (individual packages or crates) with a declared value of $3.5 million. These figures are based on "wildlife declaration forms or from official documents reporting seized, abandoned, or returned shipments" (Gaski and Johnson, 1994, p. 8).

Since so much wildlife trafficking goes undetected, it is virtually impossible to develop more accurate statistics. However, from this limited and underreported data, 60 percent of all recorded traffic was shipped via Hong Kong, most of it originating in mainland China. Of the 1.8 million medicinal items intercepted, about 30 percent (or $1.4 million worth) had ingredients from protected or endangered species and were "abandoned by the importer, refused clearance, or seized by enforcement officials" (Gaski and Johnson, 1994, p. 9).

The aforementioned five plants (ginseng, Chinese magnolia, eucommia, astragalus, and *Achyranthes bidentata*) are good examples of rare, vulnerable, and threatened species used in TCM. By sorting through publications such as *Prescription for Extinction* by Gaski and Johnson, Import Alert bulletins from the Food and Drug Administration, as well as various alternative medicine Web sites, it was possible to identify more than 400 patented Chinese remedies in which one or more of these plants were used or claimed to be used, though the formulas and ingredient claims have been scientifically verified in fewer than 20 percent of the 400 products. These insufficient data leave a great deal unknown about North American trade in these items, but are a strong indicator that such traffic is a growth market worth millions of dollars.

THE TRADE IN BEAR PARTS

Undoubtedly, the most dramatic example of endangered wildlife being threatened by the increased use of TCM is the exploitation of various bear species. Bear parts, especially bear bile, have for centuries been prescribed and used in TCM; primarily for the treatment of biliary stone disease, kidney stones, and gallbladder ailments.

The World Wildlife Fund publication *International Wildlife Trade* reports that, like most of the world's large carnivores, bear populations are declining due to habitat loss and hunting (Hemley, 1994, p. 39). Bears are hunted for sport, but also for body parts, especially their gallbladders. The breakdown of wildlife law enforcement in many of the former Soviet republics is causing serious decline in those bear populations. The major markets are China, South Korea, and Taiwan, which increasingly import bear parts from North American sources as well. Gallbladders, paws, claws, teeth, and fur are the desired parts. Bear paw soup is priced at more than $1,000 per bowl in Taiwanese restaurants where clientele seek rare and endangered species as entrees. "A desiccated gallbladder will sell for $15 in Idaho, $1,500 in Hawaii and will command $55,000 in Korea" (Espinoza, Shafer, and Hagey, 1993, p. 1363).

Medical research accumulated since 1901 has identified the unique bile acid found in bears as ursodeoxycholic acid or UDCA (also known as Urso). The only species, other than bears, known to have an appreciable or significant portion of UDCA in its bile acid is the nutria. Therefore, the Western scientific view would hypothesize that if bear bile has unique therapeutic properties, it would be due to UDCA, the only significant chemical distinction between bear bile samples and bile samples of other species.

UDCA (or Urso) is approved in the United States to treat and dissolve gallstones. In Japan, it is sold for the treatment of hepatitis, cirrhosis, jaundice, and bile duct diseases. Research in the United States on the use of UDCA shows "the greatest improvement in liver tests occur in those that are most abnormal" (Achord, 1990, p. 1091). In other words, UDCA has been shown effective (though in no sense curative) only in the most advanced cases of disease.

A very thorough laboratory analysis of bile acids in gallbladder bile obtained from "six species of bears (Ursidae), the Giant panda, the Red panda, and eleven related carnivores" was jointly conducted by staff of the Department of Medicine, University of California, San Diego; National Fish and Wildlife Forensics Laboratory, Ashland, Oregon; and Harvard Medical School, and was reported in the *Journal of Lipid Research* in 1993 (Hagey et al.,

1993). The sample included ninety-eight Ursidae, including twenty-three obtained from mainland Chinese bear farms where bears are caged and steadily "milked" for bile acid. Additionally, twenty samples of "bear bile" capsules were purchased from Chinese pharmacies. Also, a small amount of dried "bear bile" being held as criminal evidence, originating in Asia and confiscated by U.S. authorities, was analyzed.

The laboratory results from the capsules and the confiscated "bear bile" were especially relevant to the overall question of the efficacy of TCM and herbal medicines being sold in the United States. In all twenty samples of capsules, the major constituent was pig bile, not UDCA. Of the dried "bear bile" originating from Asia, only 3 percent contained UDCA; the rest contained dried pig bile (Hagey et al., 1993).

To date, this is the best biochemical study available on the medicinal properties of bear bile potions and, by implication, on the likely effectiveness of such natural remedies. For the detached observer, it is not compelling evidence of the therapeutic effect of this trusted TCM remedy. It should raise serious questions in the minds of alternative medicine users as to just what they are consuming and how effective it is. However, for the many TCM and alternative medicine users who value anecdotal testimony and traditional knowledge over laboratory results, it will not seem so conclusive.

In short, the illegal market value of bear parts will inevitably lead to the further decline or extinction of the world's bear populations so long as bear gallbladders are perceived by hundreds of millions of people as being of medicinal value and so long as such traditional beliefs are more strongly acted upon than are scientific facts. The scientific research indicates that only the polar bear, brown bear, and especially the American black bear have significant levels of UDCA. Yet the traditional association of bear gallbladders with curative powers will mean that all bear populations will continue to be harvested for their gallbladders.

The power of nonscientific beliefs also means that the consumers of bogus potions largely composed of pig bile will continue to be "cured" by these concoctions. Indeed, if scientific data were valued by the users, it would seem easy to sell UDCA derived from the gall of the relatively plentiful nutria instead of that of endangered bears. Similarly, the fact that UDCA is most effective in treating liver problems in advanced stages of disease will not prevent those with only minor ailments from buying and using "bear bile" potions.

In fact, the bogus science and absurd folklore associated with bear bile is still growing. In 1998, a poacher was arrested in Oregon as part of a gang charged with killing twenty-eight black bears, gutting them for their gallbladders, chopping off the paws, and leaving the remaining carcasses. While under arrest, he volunteered his own medical insights. Apparently you can get quite a headache from shooting bears, but luckily, fresh bear bile is a sure cure for throbbing heads. "It's bitter as hell. You've got to pretty well grit your teeth to take it," said the sixty-five-year-old retiree. "But I guarantee, it does make you feel better" (Greimel, 1998, p. 5). Surely, in this politically correct era of acknowledging all folk wisdom, we are allowed to recognize folk idiocy as well. The consumption of liquids straight from freshly killed animals is also a great way for new diseases to be transmitted from species to species. The illegal killing of bears is a million-dollar industry supported by traditional lore and beliefs that are extremely resistant to logical proof.

APHRODISIACS

The use of wildlife parts in aphrodisiacs is a widely reported issue closely related to the previous topic. The myth of the aphrodisiacal potency of compounds made from bear penis, tiger penis, and rhino horn is more spurious, anecdotal, and scientifically laughable than the tradition of the medicinal qualities of such remedies. (The use of rhino horn in aphrodisiacs is largely restricted to Middle Eastern and African regions.)

The bear, tiger, rhino, and deer populations have a sixteenth-century alchemist, who assumed the sobriquet of Paracelsus, to thank for being highly prized for their genitalia and/or horns. Paracelsus, otherwise known to his friends as Theophrastus Bombast von Hohenheim, is credited with the formulation of the "doctrine of signatures." It is among the sillier bits of folk wisdom to survive in some schools of contemporary herbal thought. The doctrine of signatures proposes that the appearance, shape, and/or color of a plant (or other substance) is a clue to how it may be used medically. In keeping with his time, Paracelsus theorized that some sort of astrological influences imprint on a plant's shape, color, or texture; thus the sensitive observer could determine its potential medical use.

By this shaky logic, quaking aspen *(Populus tremuloides)* was deemed good for treating palsy. Of St. John's wort, Paracelsus wrote, "The holes in the leaves mean that this herb helps all inner and outer orifices of the skin. The blooms rot in the form of blood, a sign that it is good for wounds and shall be used where flesh has to be treated" (Wilkinson, 1997, p. 37).

By similar reasoning, aphrodisiac aficionados conclude that the shapes of deer antlers, rhino horns, and the various penis ingredients of aphrodisiacs indicate a power that surely manifests itself as an erection.

To give him his due, Paracelsus was a man of his time, and did make more valid contributions to the foundation of early medicine. So there is no satisfaction to be taken in beating, or berating, a dead alchemist, but the modern supporters of the doctrine of signatures hardly deserve respect.

Aphrodisiacs reside in the realm of fantasy, not pharmacology, yet the environmental consequences are starkly real. The bear, tiger, and rhino populations are being decimated by poaching for such uses. Recent counts place the world tiger population at less than 3,000 and rhinos at under 11,000, while the largest bear population is the North American black bear at about 600,000. No rational argument will prevent the aphrodisiac trade from continuing and contributing to the path of extinction for these great beasts. Aside from the mass distribution of Viagra molded into the shapes of bear penis, tiger penis, and rhino horn for the Asian and Middle-Eastern markets, there is little hope. Absurd as it sounds, this might be more effective than any attempt at rational discourse with the clientele of traditional aphrodisiacs.

The myth of the naturalness of TCM literally feeds on the plants and animals harvested for its potions and remedies. The argument that herbal remedies at least do no harm rings hollow in this context. The endangered flora and fauna are evidence to the contrary.

BEAR FARMS AND PARKS

One remedial response to the international black market in bear parts is as grisly as the problem. Bear farms in China and in South Korea have sprung up as entrepreneurs try to further capitalize on this market opportunity. The mainland Chinese government encourages this type of enterprise as a means of helping to meet demand for bear bile and parts without relying on foreign sources. In these operations, bears are "milked" for bile via surgically implanted milking devices. The lives of these caged creatures are unsurprisingly nasty, brutish, and short. Details of the actual farm operations are carefully guarded information kept quiet by the Chinese not because of their gruesomeness but because the Chinese, fearing market competition, think others would want to replicate their industry (Mills, 1992, p. 42).

The Japanese prefer to keep bears in "parks" that are presented as tourist and entertainment attractions. Many of the bears have been trained to ride bikes, dance, and perform various anthropomorphic amusements for the paying visitors. These parks also have high mortality rates, as reflected in the small tins of bear meat and gallbladders sold on the premises. At least one park is reported to allow visitors who can afford the price to pick out a bear, have it slaughtered, and take away the gallbladder and choice parts (Mills and Servheen, 1991, pp. 28-30).

Conservation: Ethical or Utilitarian?

The repugnance for bear farms and bear parks felt by many Westerners is based in a moral view of environmentalism. Many Western environmentalists approach conservation and the protection of species as a moral and ethical responsibility of humans. This attitude teaches that the human species, as the top of the food chain, should practice a stewardship wherein humans are responsible to the great chain of being that is subject to our power and that we must protect the diversity of life not just for utilitarian reasons but because it is the moral or ethical thing to do. In other words, there is an attitude in Western culture that humans have a spiritual bond as well as a utilitarian connection to other life forms.

This view is rooted in precepts of European religion and philosophy, and it is not necessarily part of most Asian conservation themes. In Chinese societies, such as mainland China, Taiwan, and overseas Chinese communities, the utilitarian view of animal life prevails. This view teaches that any creature that "has its back to the sun" exists to satisfy human needs. So the justification for the practice of conservation is simply to ensure that useful species survive in numbers great enough to satisfy those human needs.

In China, the one obvious exception to this is the giant panda, now found, in nature, only in central China. (Once taxonomically categorized as distinct from bear species, the giant panda is now generally classified as a bear subspecies.) Perhaps 1,100 remain living in the wild, though poaching continues since a panda pelt can sell for $100,000. This "cute and cuddly" and uniquely Chinese creature has been used by the Chinese government to symbolize the cuddly side of the People's Republic. A sort of "panda diplomacy," in which pandas are doled out to various national zoos around the world, is one means by which mainland China has been able to project a humane image, even during periods of heightened political tensions. Thus, the Chinese government has wisely taken the view that the panda is of value in itself, and not just for its pelt and gallbladder.

But the rest of the bear species and other wildlife are protected only to be sure that they continue to be available for human use. A World Wildlife Fund scientist with years of experience in China says, "For the Chinese, conservation has entirely a utilitarian end. That is, you need to make sure there are bears somewhere—not necessarily in the wild—in order for you to continue to have gall. But that's about as far as it goes" (Mills, 1992, p. 42). So from the perspective of this utilitarian-based conservation, keeping a caged bear in a milking farm is as good a conservation practice as helping a bear to live in the wild.

Generally, people living on the edge of subsistence do not develop emotional relationships with the animals around them. A certain level of affluence is necessary before ethical relationships can be extended to nonhumans. Currently, such a view is spreading in much of Asia. For example, the Hong Kong action-film star Jackie Chan has begun to promote the Asian Conservation Awareness Program on the Internet. Jackie's home page asks his fans to talk to their older relatives and traditional Asians:

> Let's show the world that Asians do care about wildlife and that we're not prepared to sit back while these animals are wiped out, because of greed and ignorance. . . . Ask them to think first. Do they really want to be responsible for the cruel killing of an individual animal and to contribute to the extinction of the species? Don't they know that there are herbal alternatives to endangered species in traditional Chinese medicine? And do they really need that endangered

species product? No, in this day and age, there are always alternatives. There is no excuse. So please persuade them not to, for the animals' sake. (Message from Jackie Chan, <http://www.jackiewild.com>)

As an Asian superstar, Jackie Chan can speak more critically of traditional practices than can non-Asians. However, he is risking his popularity by making such an unambiguous statement and should be given credit for it. Some Asians who advocate that Asian nations and leaders must assert "Asian values" may label Chan's advocacy as proof of his "Westernization" and "neocolonialist" sentiment, but his is still a welcome voice bringing attention to a valid issue.

It is worth noting that the slaughter of bears for body parts is not objectionable solely by European or Western values. Recently, several native Canadian tribes established the First Nations Environmental Network. Their statement labels the poaching and hunting of black bears for "their gallbladders, genitalia and paws, which are used in Asian traditional medicine" as "morally and spiritually offensive to First Nation values" (Bear Watch, <http://www.bearwatch.org>).

GINSENG: POACHING OR HARVESTING?

The brutality of bear hunting and the misery of caged bears being milked for bile acid vividly illustrate a dramatic and emotional example of an endangered species further threatened by the demands for TCM and alternative medicine ingredients. Our reaction to the threats to plant species is less likely to be as passionate, but the environmental impact is much the same for several species of flora. John Garrison, a park ranger in Great Smoky Mountains National Park, is quoted as saying, "I firmly believe that ginseng poaching is our biggest threat in the park. I used to think it was bear poaching, but I think ginseng is potentially higher" (La Pierre, 1994, p. 36).

The poaching or harvesting of wild plants (often called "wild-crafting") from national and state parks and forests is a growing problem as the use of natural remedies increases. The same is probably equally true on privately held lands. Over 140 plant species found in park lands now have some market value as elements in natural remedies. Even plants such as lady's slipper and bloodroot are being dug from parks to be sold.

American ginseng *(Panax quinquefolius)* is used in many of the same medicinal remedies as Asian ginseng *(Panax ginseng)*. Wild-growing ginseng continues to be pillaged from state and national parks even though both American and Asian ginseng are now commonly cultivated in large quantities. For example, in 1992 over $10 million worth of wild ginseng was detected being illegally exported from the United States. Wild-growing plants are poached because many herbalists (both Asian and American) believe that naturally grown plants are more potent than culti-vated ones. This subjective belief keeps the wild ginseng market alive despite the easy availability of farmed ginseng. Again due to the logic of the doctrine of signatures, the "human shaped" roots are thought to be especially potent and bring the highest prices, sometimes thousands of dollars for a single root.

Due to this nonrational preference for the wild over the do-mesticated, theft from public and private lands persists even though American ginseng has been farmed for export since the 1890s. A pioneer in this enterprise, A. R. Harding, wrote in 1908 in reference to his exports to the Asian market, "—our orders for dry Ginseng root have been as high as one thousand pounds at a single order" (Harding, 1972, p. 40).

Harding commented that the Chinese preferred the wild gin-seng to the cultivated, though he, as a cultivator, held the opinion that there was no difference between the two and no way to distinguish one from the other except that the cultivated roots were usually the larger. Harding's 1908 text, *Ginseng and Other*

Medicinal Plants, is a classic of the field and, in the vernacular of the time, includes this ode to ginseng:

> Ginseng is the best and most potent of cordials, of stimulants, of tonics, of stomachics, cardiacs, febrifuges, and, above all, will best renovate and reinvigorate failing forces. It fills the heart with hilarity while its occasional use will, it is said, add a decade of years to the ordinary human life. (Harding, 1972, p. 50)

A 1992 Chinese reference states more simply of *Panax ginseng,* "This species is of important economic value as a tonic for prolonging man's life" (Fu Li-kuo, 1992, p. 178). Note that the emphasis is put on its' proven economic value rather than its debated medicinal value. Ginseng's contribution to longevity remains largely based in anecdotal evidence and folk wisdom, but this folk wisdom has made ginseng an international staple crop, nearly as important to the world economy as coffee, tea, and tobacco.

In some TCM lore, Asian ginseng is thought to have heating qualities, while American ginseng is described as cooling. However, there is no consistent explanation for why these different food properties would come from the similar ginsenosides that are found in both species. This distinction is not consistently drawn and seems especially confusing now that both *Panax ginseng* and *Panax quinquefolius* are cultivated in Asia and sometimes used interchangeably by careless manufacturers.

It should be noted that the term "ginseng" is loosely applied to several other plant species, in addition to *Panax ginseng* and *Panax quinquefolius.* In the *China Plant Red Data Book,* funded by the China National Environment Protection Agency, another species, *Panax zingiberensis,* is mentioned, but this species is not listed in any other reference sources on ginseng. *Panax pseudo-ginseng* is also widely used in Asia, and its ginsenoside content is nearly identical to that found in *Panax ginseng.* Eleuthero, not even in the same genus as true ginsengs, is called Siberian ginseng. As that common name suggests, it grows in the northern extremes of Asia. It is quite abundant and cheaper in cost, but in no way the pharmacological equivalent of true ginseng. It, and other false ginsengs, only add to the confusion surrounding the medical efficacy of ginseng. The growing popularity and financial potential of ginseng products has resulted in several nonrelated plants being sold under names such as American red ginseng, red desert ginseng, and Brazilian ginseng; they have no ginsenoside content and no proven medical efficacy. The litany of fake ginsengs only adds to the confusion and conflicting results associated with this herb (Foster and Tyler, 1999, pp. 187-193).

The commercial success of ginseng and its worldwide popularity has resulted in a tremendous amount of information and at least an equal amount of misinformation. Scientific analysis places ginseng among the class of agents called adaptogens, which "are reputed to increase the body's resistance to physical, chemical, and biological stressors" (Schulz, Hänsel, and Tyler, 1998, p. 269). In other words, ginseng seems to relieve the symptoms of stress. In today's world, stress seems pandemic, and, therefore, ginseng is popularly viewed as a panacea. The scientific literature on ginseng includes dozens of clinical studies involving thousands of subjects. Some of the results are summarized in *Rational Phytotherapy:*

[S]ubjects in 13 of the studies (1572 cases) showed improvements in mood while on treatment with the ginseng preparation. Seventeen studies (846 cases) also demonstrated improvements in physical performance. Improved intellectual performance was reported in 11 studies, and improvements in various metabolic parameters were noted in another 10 studies. All of the studies emphasized the absence or near absence of side effects relating to ginseng therapy. There was only one reported instance of tachycardia. The results were statistically evaluated in only about half the studies. On the whole, it is unlikely that the design and content of these studies would conform to current scientific standards. (Schulz, Hänsel, and Tyler, 1998, p. 273)

Thus, there are clinical results indicating that ginseng probably will help a person deal with certain stress symptoms and that, having virtually no side effects, it at least will not hurt the user. This type of scientific conclusion can and has been used by the popular press and commercial interests to turn ginseng into the answer to all ailments, especially as broadly defined a problem as stress. As a result, ginseng has been overpromoted and overused.

Legal export from the United States now exceeds fifty tons annually, the primary markets being Hong Kong, Singapore, and Taiwan (Fitzgerald, 1989, p. 299). In the Asian markets, it is used primarily as a metabolic stimulant and to regulate blood pressure, though, like so many Asian panaceas, it is also thought by many to be an aphrodisiac.

Ginseng: Purity and Potency?

The subjective nature of the debate over the efficacy of wild versus domestic ginseng, and Chinese versus American ginseng, becomes even more murky when considering a report that the Chinese government's State Administration of Traditional Chinese Medicine is now concerned over the growing number of Chinese TCM products containing "fake American ginseng." According to a UPI news release reported on the Internet, the Chinese are now cultivating American ginseng because it is "faster growing" and of "higher potency." However, the Chinese are worried that "counterfeit" American ginseng products manufactured in China are reducing the quality of Chinese products and exports (<http://www. Acupuncture.com>).

This report implies that there is little certainty whether an American ginseng product produced in China is, in fact, American or Chinese ginseng or a blend of the two or, in some cases, ginseng at all. It also suggests that cultivated American ginseng is considered more potent than wild ginseng, at least when processed in China.

All of the quality control issues that apply to any product made from herbs are compounded in ginseng. The number of "true" ginseng species plus the various fake ginsengs and the lack of regulation on many Asian suppliers results in a proliferation of very dubious ginseng products.

Regardless whether Asian or American, wild or domestic, the quality most valued by herbalists everywhere in ginseng and all other herbs is purity. The matter of purity has up to now essentially been a good faith assumption made by users that herbs, being nature's produce, are uncontaminated by chemical additives.

In May 1998, a company called PharmaPrint Inc. reported to the FDA that it had received shipments of raw ginseng root containing the fungicide quintozene, or pentrachloronitrobenzene (PCNB). PharmaPrint publicly rejected this shipment to focus maximum attention on its commitment to quality control. In all likelihood, poor quality and contaminated bulk supplies of herbs are widespread problems, with other manufacturers also receiving raw ginseng and other raw herbs containing chemical contaminants.

In addition to raising the issue of contaminants, laboratory analyses of ginseng products have shown wide variation in the levels of ginsenosides, the compounds in ginseng roots that are the active ingredients so far as any biological effects. A *Consumer Reports* study concluded that ginsenoside content "varied greatly among ten brands of ginseng" (*Consumer Reports,* 1995, p. 699). Other studies show similar results. However, even the research testing ginseng product quality is confounded by the fact that many products contain fake ginsengs and therefore have little or no ginsenoside content. In other words, products containing only fake ginsengs will show no ginsenoside content, while the products made from true ginseng species may also vary greatly in ginsenoside content.

The business goal of PharmaPrint, as well as many other producers of herbal products, is to develop a line of herbal products so standardized in content and potency that it could meet FDA standards for over-the-counter drugs. Such products are now in the development stage. PharmaPrint has negotiated with American Home products to use its Centrum brand name in this enterprise. Major pharmaceutical manufacturers offering similar lines of herbal products include Bayer and Warner-Lambert (<http://www.fast.quote.com/fg/companyresearch2/news?story>).

In the United States, ginseng is pharmacologically classified as an adaptogen, which helps the body accommodate stress. Like nearly all products thought to relieve stress, it is frequently overused, to the extent that an article in the *Journal of the American Medical Association* has identified "ginseng abuse syndrome" as an ailment in itself (Siegel, 1979, pp. 1614-1615). This study of ginseng abuse was, however, badly flawed by the lack of evidence about the ginsenoside content of products being used and overused (Castleman, 1990, pp. 23-24). About all that can really be concluded from this study is that self-prescribing, overdosing consumers can abuse anything.

Chapter 4

The Economic Growth and Social Acceptance of Alternative/Herbal Medicines in the United States

The World Health Organization reports that 80 percent of the world's population uses herbal medicine as part of their regular health care (Strohecker, 1994, p. 257). Ironically, in the United States, most such herbal remedies by law are sold not as medicines, but as "dietary supplements," a food category. When I started this study, I had a general sense that more Americans were buying and using nontraditional or alternative forms of medicine. Now I am surprised when I find a person who can say, "No, I've never used herbal remedies or supplements, and I never will." Nearly everyone who finds out that I am studying this topic can offer me an account of his or her own interest in or use of some form of alternative medical/nutritional treatment or product. Finding someone who has never used any such products is more difficult than finding a regular user.

In 1998, the "top ten" best-selling herbal supplements were echinacea, St. John's wort, ginkgo biloba, garlic, saw palmetto, Asian ginseng, goldenseal, aloe, Siberian ginseng, and valerian. These ten then accounted for nearly 55 percent of all U.S. sales. For 1998, the combined retail sales for herbal remedies totaled $3.87 billion. The fastest growing market segment was "in the mass market (supermarket, drug, and mass merchandise) increasing at an annualized rate of over 100 percent" (Brevort, 1998, p. 33).

The consumer behavior associated with herbal and "natural" products, however, is not so straightforward. On the one hand, most herbal remedy users believe that herbs and their compounds or extracts can heal, cure, or invigorate. Yet they consume herbs as though they are harmless, because their assumption is that if it is "natural," it can do no harm and can be taken in any combination or quantity.

Yet it is known that certain herbs—for example, comfrey and germander—can cause liver toxicity, that the herbal dieting ingredient ma huang (ephedra) is linked to several deaths by heart failure, and that some herbs can induce abortion. Also, for many herbal products, especially those imported from Asia, there is no assurance of purity of ingredient, quality, basic manufacturing hygiene, or protection from adulteration by pesticides.

SAFETY AND EFFICACY

Often the only testing of imported herbs is the spot testing of illegal imports confiscated by the U.S. Fish and Wildlife Service. These limited tests have shown the presence of toxic substances such as arsenic and mercury. Both arsenic and mercury tend to bioconcentrate when taken internally thus low dosages taken over long periods of time can accumulate to toxic levels. For centuries, realgar (arsenic sulfide) and cinnabar (mercury) have been included in the traditional Chinese pharmacopoeia. Both realgar and cinnabar are normal ingredients, especially in products that claim to be tiger bone or rhinoceros horn compounds (U.S. Fish and Wildlife Service, <http://www.fws.gov/r9dia/asian/html>).

The California Department of Health Services also has conducted a limited study "to screen imported Asian patent medicines for undeclared pharmaceuticals and heavy metal contamination" (Ko, 1998, p. 847). Of 260 Asian patent medicines collected from

California retail stores, eighty-three (32 percent) contained un-declared pharmaceuticals and/or heavy metals (lead, arsenic, mercury). The remaining products "can not be assumed to be safe and free of toxic ingredients, in view of their batch-to-batch inconsistency" (p. 847).

The FDA generates Import Alerts, periodical bulletins, for concerned government agencies, such as U.S. Customs and Immigration and the U.S. Fish and Wildlife Service, on medicines being brought into the United States that do not conform to FDA standards. Habitually, Chinese herbal medicines are among the main violators. Most of the violations have been detected in air mail shipments to health food stores, Asian food stores, and Asian pharmacies. These violations include products found by the FDA to:

- contain undeclared drug substances;
- have inadequate labeling directions for use;
- contain an unapproved new drug;
- contain undeclared metals/metalloids;
- contain potentially toxic ingredients;
- contain specially regulated ingredients (codeine, opium powder, cannabis seed); and
- make unproved treatment claims for serious medical conditions (Import Alert #6610, <http://www.fda.gov/ora/fiars/ora_import_ia6610.html>).

Some of the most dubious TCM remedies are shipped from China and distributed via mail order companies in the United States. These products range from the relatively harmless baldness cures to aphrodisiacs to spurious cancer cures. A California mail order operation offers remedies such as:

Remedy	Ingredient	Claim
Perfect Manhood Pill	unknown	cures impotence, nocturnal emission, lumbago, white hair and beard, frequent urination
Red Peach Hair Tonic	unknown	has an extraordinary effect on prevention of alopecia (thin hair and bald head)
Venus Men's Towel	unknown	can prolong erection and increase sensation, especially for men suffering from premature ejaculation
China No. 1 Tian Xian Liquid	unknown	an efficient remedy for curing cancer, especially in the middle and late stages of illness

Source: Attachment A, Import Alert #6610, <http//www.fda.gov/ora/fiars/ora>.

One of the most notorious examples of TCM potions adulterated with controlled substances is the well-documented Black Pearls. Variously called Black Pearls, Chiufong Toukawan, Cow's Head, and Tung Shueh, they have been sold for a variety of illnesses from arthritis to sexual impotence. They were widely distributed in California, Texas, and throughout the southwestern states. They are associated with at least four deaths. In various forms and batches they contained "a variety of controlled substances such as chlordiazepoxide (a benzodiazepine), betamethasone, dexamethasone, methyl testosterone, prednisolone, and theophylline" (Wesdock, 1998, p. 7). Normally, tranquilizers, steroids, diuretics, and male hormones are not prescribed in one drug for women with arthritis. Fraud and quackery are possible in all medical fields, but the herbal market is especially susceptible to such abuses.

Even with legal and "harmless" herbal products, there may be no proof of the presence of the claimed "active ingredient." Feverfew is an herb that can help treat migraine, due to its ingredient parthenolide. A limited study of a few (sixteen) of the feverfew products sold in Toronto yielded this result:

- Nine products met the label claim of the presence and concentration of parthenolide
- Five products contained parthenolide but not in the claimed concentration
- Two products contained no parthenolide (Market Place, <http://www.tv.cbc.ca/market/files/herbdrugs.html>)

Questions of safety and efficacy have to be addressed one by one as new dietary supplements come on the market and as older ones suddenly become popular and used widely enough for side effects to begin to appear. Sleeping Buddha, a sleep and relaxation dietary supplement made in China and marketed by a Canadian-based distributor, was another recent example. It was withdrawn after the FDA determined that it contained prescription-strength estazolam, a sedative of the benzodiazepine group, which has side effects including potential fetal damage (Medwatch, <http://www.pharminfo.com/medwatch/mwrpt36.html>).

The "fen-phen" controversy was more widely reported. As the risk to cardiac valves associated with these various fenfluramine-phentermine-based dieting pills became known, the FDA required more stringent labeling and monitoring of use. Soon, many "natural" herbal alternatives came on the market. In nearly all herbal fen-phen products, the herbal ingredient is ma huang, the herbal source of ephedrine. The alkaloid ephedrine is an amphetamine-like compound that can act upon the heart and nervous system in potentially dangerous ways. The herbal fen-phen products not containing ma huang were found to contain 5-hydroxytryptophan (about which the FDA has now issued a warning), which is nearly identical to L-tryptophan. L-tryptophan was taken off the market in 1990 when it was linked to 1,500 cases (including thirty-eight deaths) of a rare blood disorder called eosinophilia-mylagia syndrome (EMS).

Because of their amphetamine-like effects upon the nervous system, ma huang-based products are also popular with long-distance truckers, who take them to stay awake, and with others who seek a natural, herbal alternative to what they think of as euphoria-inducing drugs.

Euphoria is literally a state of mind, and in this situation we are talking about people who choose to interpret stresses upon the nervous system as a state of heightened consciousness. In TCM, ma huang is often used to relieve common cold symptoms by inducing sweating, or to "open" the lungs of asthma sufferers, and to promote urination. In doing so, ma huang may elevate blood pressure and cause arrhythmia and "restlessness." For highly suggestible "euphoria" seekers, apparently these side effects can be interpreted as increased energy and heightened sensuality. As a consequence, many ma huang products have been marketed as euphoria-producing alternatives to street drugs.

After a recent death due to overdose, the State of New York has banned the sale of the following ma huang-based products: Ultimate Xphoria, Cloud 9, Herbal Ecstasy, Euphoria, X Tablets, Legal Weed, Rave Energy, HerbalXTC, Hextasy, Ecstasy, Buzz Tablets, Planet X, Fungalore, Naturally High, The Drink, Fukola Cola Brain Wash, Love Potion #69, Black Lemonade, and Brainalizer (Acupuncture.com, <http://www.acupuncture.com>).

Fukola Cola Brain Wash and its competitors have very few defenders even on the various "health freedom" Web sites. However, the matter of red yeast-bearing Cholestin is a far more controversial case, finding great support on these Web sites. Pharmanex Co. produces Cholestin, a dietary supplement made from rice fermented with red yeast, which is imported from China. (Red is the variant of the yeast, not a comment on the politics of the source.) Cholestin is sold nationwide in 37,000 stores, including Wal-Mart, as a dietary supplement that "promotes healthy cholesterol" (Acupuncture.com, <http://www.acupuncture.com>).

The FDA does not question the effectiveness of Cholestin in promoting healthy cholesterol. On the contrary, in this case, the

FDA wanted Cholestin categorized as a drug rather than a dietary supplement and went to court to pursue such a ruling.

The FDA position was that the fermented red yeast contains lovastatin, which is an active ingredient in cholesterol-lowering prescription drugs; therefore, the Pharmanex Co. should be required to do the necessary research to get Cholestin approved as a drug. The FDA argued that Pharmanex is using the 1994 Dietary Supplement Health and Education Act as a means to avoid the drug-approval process.

The Pharmanex counter position was that red yeast rice is a food and therefore Cholestin is a dietary supplement which just happens to "promote healthy cholesterol."

The U.S. District Court of Utah, Central Division, handed down its judgment on June 16, 1998. It ruled in favor of Pharmanex, that Cholestin could be regulated by the FDA only as a dietary supplement, not as a drug. That is where the Cholestin issue now remains.

The larger question here is: What is the difference between an FDA-approved drug and an herbal product which contains naturally occurring chemicals that have the potency and efficacy of drugs? The final legal answer to this question is ultimately worth billions of dollars.

The Cholestin ruling was significant in itself to Pharmanex, but in the long run it was only the tip of an iceberg. The name of this iceberg is nutraceuticals or functional foods. More and more major food companies such as Kellogg, Nabisco, Nestlé, General Mills, and others see a new market in functional foods.

This is a further blurring of the line between foods and drugs. Examples include "calcium in Tropicana orange juice, and echinacea in Fresh Samantha drinks; Stoneyfield yogurt has *L. reuteri* bacteria to protect against *Salmonella* and *E. coli* 0157:H7. Psyllium has been added to cereal, frozen entrees, bread and pasta in Kellogg's Ensemble line. As functional foods have moved from natural-food stores to supermarkets, sales have reached $17 billion" (Burros, 1998, p. B12). The ultimate question remains: Are these and future forms of nutraceuticals really foods, dietary supplements, or drugs?

HERBAL POLITICS

This is both a legal question and a political question. At this writing, the FDA is seeking to revise its rules regarding permissible labeling claims in order to address this question. The original deadline for public input on new proposals was August 27, 1998. Senator Orrin Hatch, R-Utah, sought and received an extension of the deadline to allow more public input. Both herbal Web sites and health supplement stores are now gearing up to promote letter-writing campaigns by their users. Form letters and talking points on health freedom, medical choice, herbal alternatives, overregulation of medicine, and the growth of global pharmaceutical companies are available at the stores and on the Internet. Some encourage rather overripe prose, such as:

> We are *ON* to your little shell game, FDA! We have *TAKEN NOTICE* of the despicable efforts . . . to force the global harmonization of laws governing the manufacture and sale of herbal products, just as we are **ALSO** *enraged* by the German Codex Proposal to restrict our access to only RDA levels of vitamins and minerals! . . . *BACK OFF, FDA, OBEY THE LAW.* (International Advocates for Health Freedom, <http://www.iahf.com/fdacomments.html>)

The organization responsible for this prose is the International Advocates for Health Freedom, a legislative advocacy group based in Hollywood, Florida. Its self-proclaimed mission is to aid the public in understanding the "MACRO view of what we are facing in America, by gaining sufficient awareness to be able to SEE the pharmaceutical take over pattern!" (IAHF would really have something to fear if the international pharmaceutical conspiracy began to regulate the use of uppercase, bold, and italic fonts. Probably all Web site information should be accompanied by a warning to the effect that it can be hazardous to your mental health.)

The rhetoric of paranoia and persecution used by so many alternative medicine advocates is unfortunate and self-defeating. It undermines valid concerns over the growth of a pharmaceutical monopoly by a few international drug companies and the subsequent reduction of consumer choice. These are real issues that should be topics of rational public discussion.

After all, the 1994 Dietary Supplement Health and Education Act is a political document as well as a regulatory law. Senator Orrin Hatch, a major author of this law, is very attentive to the many Utah-based dietary supplement companies, which do $2 billion in annual sales. According to the Center for Responsive Politics, from 1991 to 1996, health products companies contributed $277,000 to his campaigns (Japsen, 1998, pp. 1, 19).

Senator Hatch, Congressman Peter DeFazio, and Senator Thomas Harkin are valued allies of the alternative medicine and health freedom lobbies. Such political influence on approved medicine in America has a long tradition. In the 1930s Senator Royal Copeland (New York), a homeopath, lobbied successfully on behalf of homeopathic remedies.

Despite the uncertainties and potential dangers of herbal products, in both the United States and Canada any attempt to further regulate the marketing of herbal food supplements/medicines brings enormous resistance from grassroots users and from the herbal products industry. The office staff of my congressional representative confirmed that they receive some of their heaviest mail whenever any issue of alternative medicine is being debated in Congress or by a federal agency. The many herbal Web sites usually present such discussion as attacks on medical and health freedoms. One site proclaims, "The struggle for freedom of medical choice is *The* political issue of the decade" (Viable Herbal Solutions, <http://www.lef.org>).

In 1998, the herbal Web sites were extremely supportive of the Access to Medical Treatment Act, H.R. 746 (House), introduced by Oregon Congressman Peter DeFazio. Stated briefly, this bill would permit patients to be treated by any health practitioner legally sanctioned to provide professional health services in their state, with any method of medical treatment that the patient requests. *In other words, this would allow the patient to request and receive a treatment not yet approved by the FDA.*

From the viewpoint of its advocates, it would only give the patient the freedom to select appropriate treatments not yet sanctioned by the FDA. Their argument is that FDA approval of a treatment takes an average of ten years and $300 million, thus heavily favoring large pharmaceutical companies which prefer products that can be patented. Because existing species of plants and animals and their known constituents cannot normally be patented, the large drug companies rarely pursue research in such areas (Viable Herbal Solutions, <http://www.lef.org>).

From the viewpoint of orthodox health care providers and the FDA, H.R. 746 is a Pandora's box that would unleash untold quackery. Those who do not support this bill point out that it would allow a doctor or other health professional to treat people with drugs or devices unapproved by the FDA, without having to obtain an IND/DE (investigational new drug/device exemption).

Amendments to the Federal Food, Drug, and Cosmetic Act signed into law in 1997 now permit individuals with serious medical problems, for which no approved therapies are effective, to obtain experimental therapies if the manufacturer will provide them. The FDA also has a "compassionate use" program, but one still must receive FDA approval of the medical protocol.

H.R. 746 also specifies that "dangerous medical treatment" must be reported to the Secretary of Health and Human Services, while "beneficial medical treatment" is to be reported to the recently established Office of Alternative Medicine.

After the Access to Medical Treatment bill was introduced, it was referred to the House Commerce Committee, which has jurisdiction over amendments to the Federal Food, Drug, and Cosmetic Act. In August 1998, I was told by a congressional staff person that it was "unlikely this bill would be considered."

Another bill, H.R. 2868, the Consumer Health Free Speech Act, has more recently been sponsored by Congressman Ron Paul (R-Texas). The goal of this bill is to remove "food" (meaning dietary supplements) from the definition of "drug" in the 1994 Act, in order to permit dietary supplements to make therapeutic claims in their labeling. Currently the 1994 Act defines "drug" as "articles intended for use in the diagnosis, cure, mitigation, treatment, or prevention of disease in man . . ." H.R. 2868 would add three words, "other than food," changing the definition to "articles, *other than food,* intended for use in the diagnosis, cure, mitigation, treatment, or prevention of disease in man . . ." Congressman Paul's goal is to exempt all foods (especially herbs and dietary supplements) from FDA regulation. This bill also currently resides in the House Commerce Committee.

Should the Commerce Committee decide to debate this bill and make a distinction between food and dietary supplements, it would be well served by a look at the writing of Dr. Hun Young Cho, a Korean medical practitioner trained in both TCM and modern medicine:

> A food while giving a healing effect on a sick person, is a substance beneficial even to a healthy body. Medicinal substances, on the other hand, need not be taken if a person is not sick, and can be harmful when taken by a healthy person. (Cho, 1996, pp. 187-188)

Dr. Cho is often quoted by TCM and herbal advocates, and by his above distinction, dietary supplements would either be of no medical substance at all, or they should be overseen by the FDA and avoided by healthy people. This is probably not what the dietary supplements lobby had in mind.

The Access to Medical Treatment bill and the Consumer Health Free Speech bill are only two indicators of the continuing confrontation between the established and the alternative medical communities in American society. Another indicator, equally unnoticed by the general public, was the creation of the Office of Alternative Medicine (Senator Harkin being its chief sponsor), a part of whose charge is to encourage research on "unconventional medical practices." In 1991, the Congress set aside, in the fiscal year 1992 budget of the National Institute of Health, funding to create the Office of Alternative Medicine. If, as H.R. 746 directs, it is only to receive reports of "beneficial medical treatments," it should easily satisfy its charge to encourage unconventional medical practices.

The Office of Alternative Medicine has been in operation since 1992, yet most citizens are unaware of its existence. Bureaucracies grow by stealth rather than publicity, and OAM is no exception to this rule. Advocates have made the case that its lack of productivity is due to its structure rather than its mission. Thus, in 1998 Congress restructured it from an Office into a Center. As the National Center for Complementary and Alternative Medicine (NCCAM), it is empowered to directly fund its own projects. With a budget of $50 million, its research ability should be enhanced. It has now designated thirteen regional centers at various universities and institutes for alternative medical research.

The bureau's former director, Dr. Wayne Jonas, commented:

In 10 years, the Office of Alternative Medicine will be a thriving organizational entity working closely with other NIH components and federal agencies, academic centers, private organizations, and the public to facilitate quality research that integrates complementary and alternative medicine and conventional healing approaches. (Marwick, 1998, p. 1553)

What remains to be seen is whether an NCCAM can successfully move from its advocacy role to the position of generating truly objective, scientific research without alienating its political base in the alternative medicine-dietary supplements industry lobby.

For any medical remedy to be classified as a "drug" by the FDA, it must be proven safe for the user and effective against its targeted ailment by undergoing rigorous, prolonged, and expensive testing which involves double-blind research techniques. Though valid research for many herbs exists in Europe, the FDA has not accepted most of these herbal research databases. Therefore, the 1994 Dietary Supplement Act ensures that until an herbal remedy has been tested in the United States and approved by the FDA, it can be sold and advertised only as a "dietary supplement" or "health maintenance" product. Labels must make no medicinal claim and must indicate the absence of FDA drug approval. However, so long as a dietary supplement is properly labeled, the burden of proof is on the FDA to show that it is unsafe, rather than on the manufacturer to show that it is safe. This is a marketplace in which the dictum "caveat emptor" certainly applies.

Denied drug or medicinal classification, the herbal industry has learned how to rely on advertising that emphasizes the images and adjectives of "health" and "nature." Instead of research findings, these products rely on the anecdotal testimony and endorsements of users and various celebrities including some athletes who promote fitness programs. The FDA restrictions under which the herbal industry operates only makes its current growth more impressive. The dietary supplement category, though limited and confining, is a niche to which the herbal producers have successfully adapted. No wonder then that they should be alarmed by any further proposed regulation of their products when they are already defensive about their status.

Their worst fear currently takes the form of the dreaded Codex Alimentarius Commission (CAC). This arcanely named organization is perceived by the herbal community as an international conspiracy of *X-Files* proportion. One Web site (Acupuncture. com, <http://www.acupuncture.com>) has referred to it as "the greatest threat to health freedom in the world today." The CAC is a committee including 146 member nations, operating under the United Nations and the World Health Organization. Its stated purpose is to protect consumers worldwide by establishing international guidelines for food and botanical products. In 1995, the German delegation to this commission proposed a set of four guidelines for dietary supplements:

1. No vitamin, mineral, herb, etc., can be sold for prophylactic (preventive) or therapeutic use.
2. None sold as a food can exceed potency (dosage) levels set by the commission.
3. Codex regulations for dietary supplements would become binding—eliminating the escape clause within the General Agreement on Tariffs and Trade (GATT) that allows a nation to set its own standards.
4. All new dietary supplements would automatically be banned unless they go through the Codex approval process. (Acupuncture.com, <http://www.acupuncture.com>)

This is now ominously referred to on various Web sites as "the German proposal." Briefly stated, this proposal would require research-based standards of appropriate potency and dosage to be established for all herbal/dietary supplement products. These guidelines would appear to, in effect, establish daunting standards and a layer of international bureaucracy seemingly impossible for small companies to overcome before marketing a product.

This proposal is portrayed by herb users and producers as an attack on the health rights of Americans, and as a devious scheme promoted by international drug companies to make the CAC approval process so difficult and costly that only major international corporations could afford to operate in the dietary supplements market. By driving small manufacturers from the market, the handful of major international pharmaceutical companies would then take over the herbal supplements industry through the sanctioning authority of GATT and the CAC (Life Extension Foundation, <http://www.lef.org>).

HERBAL BUSINESS

In point of fact, the dietary supplements business is no longer a mom-and-pop cottage industry. Despite the demurs and cries of self-defined victimization by the dietary supplements manufacturers, the real struggle here is between big business and bigger business. As the profitability of the industry has risen, it is now attracting companies such as Celestial Seasonings Inc., Wal-Mart's private label Spring Valley, the Warner-Lambert Co., American Home Products (Centrum brand name), and the Bayer Corporation into the market. Kmart Corporation is starting a home shopping Web site, Family and Fitness, <http://www.FamilyandFitness.com>, to market vitamins, herbals, and homeopathic products online.

As far as the issue of naturalness, if a product comes in shrink-wrap, or a safety-sealed box, or a bottle with a childproof lid, it is not freshly harvested from the earth. Most dietary supplements are natural in the same sense that an automobile is a product of nature because iron ore comes from the earth. It is a manufactured industrial product, no matter how many flowers adorn the wrapper, no matter how many times the label invokes the word "nature." Herbal product companies are no longer neighborhood herbalists and healers grinding up plants from the backyard garden.

Even without the Codex Alimentarius Commission to conjure the image of a conspiratorial cabal, both users and producers of alternative medicines tend to see themselves as outsiders beset by establishment standards and attitudes. Correctly or incorrectly, many people in the United States turn to alternative health practices and remedies because they feel that mainstream medicine is not serving their health needs. In other words, the dislike and rejection of conventional medical practices may be as great a contributor to the success of alternative medicines as is the user's satisfaction with such products. Stated briefly, people are frustrated by their experience of the established medical profession and looking to alternative medicines as a solution.

A study of malpractice claims among physicians states it this way:

> Treating the whole person—the hallmark of alternative medicine—begins with actually giving the individual patient enough attention during the office visit to allow them to come into view. Alternative practitioners know this because their modalities require detailed case taking; conventional doctors may come to know this because they cannot afford the malpractice claims that result from ignoring it. (Viable Herbal Solutions, <http://www.lef.org>)

A similar conclusion was reported by a focus-group study of patient attitudes that portrayed conventional medical practice as a "confusing, expensive, unreliable and often impersonal disassembly of medical professionals and institutions" (Picker Institute, <http://www.picker.com>).

Thus, two concomitant factors are really energizing this growth of herbal/alternative medicines. The American public is rejecting current conventional medical practice as it is simultaneously embracing alternative methods. The growing use of alternative medicines calls attention to the unpopularity of the medical establishment as much, or more, than it demonstrates proof of the efficacy of alternative methods (in fact, the efficacy of alternative methods and potions remains largely unproven).

AMA AND ALTERNATIVES

The AMA is aware of this trend and in its stately, procedural fashion is trying to respond. In 1996, a detailed and reasonably balanced study on alternative medicine use was presented to the AMA by its Council on Scientific Affairs (Natural HealthLine, <http:// www.naturalhealthvillage.com/reports/council_of_sci_affairs. htm>). This report noted that of patients seeing an MD, more than one-fourth also used some form of alternative therapy; the majority of this one-fourth did not so inform the physician. The research indicated that the total number of visits to alternative practitioners (425 million) actually exceeded visits to primary care physicians (388 million). Thus the possibilities of overmedication and conflicting medication are real. The same research placed the 1990 cost to users of alternative therapies (including dietary supplements and herbal medicines) at over $10 billion, with an additional $3 billion paid by insurers and third parties.

The reasons or symptoms for which people turn to alternative therapies range from the trivial (dry hair) to the desperate (cancer). That desperation is compounded by an aimless abundance of alternative cancer therapies including acupuncture, chelation, multiple-vitamin therapy, shark cartilage, Chinese herbs, homeopathic capsules, mistletoe, and mushrooms.

It seems nonproductive to simply attribute this medical shopping to an "outbreak of irrationalism," as some AMA defenders do. Taking that approach, one should also note equally strong outbreaks of interest in better health and fitness, outbreaks of well-based skepticism toward the rushed practices of many physicians, and outbreaks of patients taking responsibility for their own health.

The 1996 AMA report does pass on the advice that doctors should keep an open mind regarding patients' views of alternative medicines, neither accepting at first glance nor rejecting out of hand their effectiveness, and avoiding an attitude of "hubris and arrogance" in regard to alternative medicines. In the report's words, "accurate, even-handed education about alternative medicine is vital."

The report recommends that the following four points be adopted as AMA policy regarding alternative therapies:

1. There is very little evidence to confirm the safety or efficacy of most alternative therapies. Much of the evidence currently known about these therapies makes it clear that many have not been shown to be efficacious. Well-designed, stringently controlled research should be done to evaluate the efficacy of alternative therapies.

(By continuing to lump a widely disparate range of therapies into one category, the AMA can continue to make this assertion. However, the qualifying words "most," "much," and "many" in this statement acknowledge that not all alternative therapies are lacking research support of their efficacy. If the AMA is sincere about formulating a new policy pertaining to alternative therapies, then it must begin to distinguish those therapies now supported by scientific research, for example, phytotherapy as regulated in Germany, from those therapies not validated by a research database.)

2. Physicians should routinely inquire about the use of alternative or unconventional therapy by their patients, and educate themselves and their patients about the state of scientific knowledge with regard to alternative therapy that may be used or contemplated.
3. Courses offered by medical schools on alternative medicine should present the scientific view of unconventional theo-

ries, treatments, and practice as well as the potential therapeutic utility, safety, and efficacy of these modalities.
4. Patients who choose alternative therapies should be educated
   as to the hazards that might result from postponing or stopping
   conventional medical treatment. (<http://www.naturalhealth
   village.com/council_of_sci_affairs>)

It should be noted that a study by D. Eisenberg and colleagues
(the data source for the Council on Scientific Affairs report) was a
telephone survey of a national sample (1,539) of adults eighteen
years and older, in 1990. The methodology was thorough and scientifically rigorous (Eisenberg et al., 1993). However, two sampling
criteria may have actually eliminated many alternative therapy users
from the sample. First, the sample was limited to households with
telephones, thus missing alternative therapy users living in shelters
and various institutional settings. Second, the sample was limited to
English speakers, which suggests that many users of TCM and
various Asian (and South American) healing therapies were underreported.

The AMA refers to the Flexner report of 1910 as the beginning
of modern medicine in America. It is, in the sense of being the
beginning of the dominance of a biologically based, disease-
focused practice of medicine, the establishment of accreditation
of medical schools based on teaching the allopathic model, and
licensing by state boards dedicated to this view of medicine.

This is also the beginning of "alternative" medicine in the
sense that all practices outside of the allopathic, disease-based
medical theory and practice then found themselves viewed as
less than legitimate. Prior to that, homeopathy, osteopathy, and
naturopathy all were practiced with relatively equal status to
allopathy. But after 1910, these medical models along with herbalism, folk remedies, chiropractic, and other less-practiced therapies found themselves grouped as unconventional medicines.

Aside from sharing this common grouping in contradistinction to the medical establishment, the alternative medicines have as many differences as they do commonalities. In addition to the relatively "homegrown" varieties of American alternatives (homeopathy, osteopathy, chiropractic, etc.), any current list must now include TCM, acupuncture, and Ayurvedic, as well as South American and Afro-Caribbean spirit healing. If there is a common theme that binds them together as a group, it would be characterized by emphases on:

1. a physical-spiritual-psychological unity through which body and mind are reciprocally influential, and capable of promoting self-healing;
2. natural therapies and herbs being considered preferable to medical technologies and drugs; and
3. the importance of diet and nutrition, based on herbs and whole foods, to health.

To an unfortunate degree, the historical relationship of AMA mainstream medicine and its alternatives has been adversarial. At the beginning of the twentieth century, as medicine was becoming a profession, it needed to police its own house in order to prevent quackery and to reward the highest standards. Both camps became defensive; the alternative models wanted to defend their own traditions, and the AMA wanted to protect its standards of practice. Now when there seem to be both reasons and means to seek a new accommodation, it is hard to break the old habits of mutual distrust.

ALTERNATIVE INSURANCE

As more patients seek an alternative to conventional medical practices and take their ailments and business to alternative practitioners, even the health insurance industry is slowly being forced to recognize the trend. In California (where all such trends seem to start), state laws, California Senate Bills 840 and 2179, require both Worker's Compensation Insurance and all group insurance plans to cover acupuncture. In Connecticut, a private insurance system called the Oxford Health Plans has extended coverage to include a broad range of alternative medicines—"reflexology, Thai [*sic*] Chi, hypnotherapy, meditation, and other body energy approaches" (Hube, 1996, p. 25). The Oxford company is even putting together a network of alternative providers that the insured may visit directly without MD referral. The reasons, according to Oxford, are "consumer demand" and "unarguable cost savings (most alternative therapies cost less than conventional treatments)" (p. 25).

The cost savings argument assumes that direct access to alternative practitioners will result in a decline in the use of conventional servers. Depending upon one's viewpoint, the good news and the bad news is that this has the effect of shifting the responsibility of diagnosis to the consumer or patient. Ultimately that may prove to be both more costly and more risky.

By now, at least twenty-five companies offer some alternative therapy coverage and many more plan to so expand their coverage. An HMO in Albuquerque is reported to cover referrals to "Mexican medicine healers." And a Seattle clinic for homeless youth has added acupuncture and naturopathic care to its services (Acupuncture.com, <http://www.acupuncture.com>). One insurer, the Alliance for Natural Health, now offers a medical insurance plan covering the following: acupuncture, alternative birthing centers and midwives, Ayurvedic medicine, bodywork and massage therapy, biofeedback, chelation therapy, chiropractic, colonic therapy, herbal medicine, homeopathic and naturopathic medicines, oriental medicine, osteopathy, nutritional counseling, and transcendental meditation (Alternative Health Insurance, <http://www.alternative-insurance.com/the%20Plan.html>).

When even insurance companies acknowledge a social trend, it can no longer be thought of as frivolous or merely a fringe element. The growth of alternative medicines is very much a part of modern medicine in America. What now seems to be developing in the United States is a "multiple-path medicine," similar to the pattern of many Asian societies, in which American patients are going to mix and match establishment and alternative remedies to suit their own perception of health.

Chapter 5

"Like Two Wings of a Bird"?

One of the fairest, most balanced discussions of the attempt to philosophically integrate TCM and Western medicine is a fifty-year-old book by a Korean doctor, Hun Young Cho, titled *Oriental Medicine: A Modern Interpretation*, translated into English by Kihyon Kim. The author intended the book primarily for a Western audience and, by writing it, hoped to cast light on the real differences, and relative strengths and weaknesses of both systems as he came to see them after years of study in both traditions. (Though the term "oriental" is no longer politically correct among many Asians and scholars of Asian culture, I will use it in regard to this book.)

Throughout the book, Cho contrasts the two medical systems by means of what he calls "critical comparisons":

Oriental Medicine	Western Medicine
1. Theory and practice are grounded in philosophy.	1. Theory and practice are grounded in physical sciences.
2. Approach is holistic.	2. Approach is analytic.
3. Defines health as the cultivation of the *internal* life force (Qi).	3. Defines health as the elimination of disease and *external* pathogens.
4. Observation of total being.	4. Investigation of the structure of matter.
5. Treats root causes.	5. Treats manifestations and symptoms.
6. Phenomenal medicine.	6. Structural medicine.
7. Study of syndromes.	7. Study of anatomy.
8. Adapts (diagnosis and treatment are individually formed).	8. Standardizes (seeks to place disease and treatment in the context of universally valid rules of science).

The specifics of these comparisons can be endlessly debated, but Cho's concern is not in the details so much as in the patterns of each medical tradition. It is also far more useful to think of these as points on a continuum rather than as dichotomous categories. In other words, Oriental medicine is not solely, but is primarily, grounded in philosophy; Western medicine is not solely, but is primarily, grounded in the physical sciences. Oriental medicine is not solely, but is primarily, holistic; Western medicine is not solely, but is primarily, analytic. And so on.

Throughout his book, the author stresses that neither system can be sincerely evaluated using the standards of only one or the other: ". . . bias cannot be avoided in discussing Oriental medicine while looking only from the perspective of Oriental medicine. Also, a biased opinion can not be avoided in discussing methods outside of Western medicine when coming from a contemporary scientific standpoint" (Cho, 1996, p. 1).

Cho writes that a true commitment to the treatment of the sick cannot afford the luxury of ideological purity, but rather necessitates a reasoned use of both systems.

> We must praise the strong points of Western medicine and at the same time supplement the weak points. In my opinion, the method of supplementation can be adopted only from Oriental medicine. . . . Western and Oriental medicine should not oppose one another. It is not a matter of which one is superior. Though the duties undertaken and the direction of contribution may differ, when looking from a wide viewpoint as a medicine, there is a feeling that Oriental and Western medicine are like two wings of a bird. When both fully communicate, then it will be possible to give the best in medical treatment. (Cho, 1996, pp. 2, 10)

MEDICINE, AUTHORITY, AND WEALTH

In addition to this plea for communication and cooperation between the two medicines, Cho makes a telling observation relevant to this study. He states that Western medicine is the medicine of authority and wealth:

> Western medicine, in contrast to Oriental medicine, is the medicine most appropriate for use by the government. For the prevention of epidemics in a country or for judicially related medical needs such as blood type, finger prints, autopsy, etc., Western medicine is most effective. That is why the support of the government has always been given to Western medicine.
>
> Those who are concerned about Oriental medicine should remember that it is always in a disadvantageous position compared to modern medicine which has formed a trinity with government authority and monetary resources. (Cho, 1996, pp. 9-10)

Certainly a modern American trinity composed of AMA-sanctioned medicine, government regulatory agencies, and industrial wealth is exactly the power complex described by so many alternative medicine advocates, as well as more detached observers. What is less clear is whether the shrill complaints of the alternative medicine/dietary supplement industry are dedicated to dismantling this complex or expanding it from a trinity into a quartet.

Asian experts and practitioners of TCM and herbal medicine stress the need in their own countries for a medical pluralism in which Western and Asian health and healing practices are both used as the illness necessitates. Perhaps this is no surprise, coming from Asian cultures in which the art of compromise is highly valued.

Here in America, hints of future compromise are emerging. Even the AMA is showing signs of learning to live with medicines not yet embraced by its sanction. The report of the Council on Scientific Affairs concludes as follows:

> Given the growing interest in alternative medicine by the public, accurate, even-handed education about alternative medicine is vital for both the public as well as for physicians, who should be familiar with unconventional therapies and be able to advise patients on their use. Sound, good quality research is needed to determine the potential benefits and avoid the risks inherent in unconventional therapy. (Acupuncture. com, <http://www.naturalhealthvillage.com/reports/council_ of_sci_affairs.htm>)

In this same spirit, in 1997, a panel of experts from the NIH endorsed the use of acupuncture for pain following dental surgery or other surgery, nausea associated with chemotherapy or pregnancy, tennis elbow, and carpal tunnel syndrome. The same panel suggested that acupuncture prescribed along with biomedical treatment could be effective in stroke rehabilitation, menstrual cramps, low back pain, and asthma. Then the panel added the caveat, "there is no evidence that confirms the theory that acupuncture's efficacy is due to the existence of Qi energy" (<http:// www.acupuncture.com/news/sam.htm>).

Often, the most strident rhetoric and extreme positions come from the converts to a cause, and alternative medicine is no exception to this truism. Some American converts to Asian medicine speak and write with an almost religious zeal. For example, here is a response to the NIH panel by a licensed acupuncturist writing on the Acupuncture.com Web site:

> Oriental medicine has a great deal to offer the Western discipline of internal medicine, perhaps more than the "pain control" applications that are finally being accepted in the Western medical community. Ten years ago, using acupuncture for muscular pain control too, was considered quite

silly. In another ten years, I hope that we'll see a greater acceptance of Oriental medicine's true genius, and that is in the area of internal medicine.

The writer goes on to advise readers that an MD with proper training can probably perform acupuncture for pain control, but that

> for anything else, it would be a really good idea to search out a practitioner who has been trained in traditional Oriental medical theory . . . to act upon the Yang in your body as well as the Yin.
>
> If there are no <u>acupuncturists practicing in your area</u> due to the <u>laws of your state</u>, then a good idea would be to seek out a school of Chinese martial arts such as Kung Fu, Tai Chi, and others. They often know of practitioners of Oriental medicine who practice "underground." There are certain legal problems with this, but sometimes pain can motivate one to seek out help wherever it can be found. (<http://www.acupuncture.com/Acup/Comparison.html>)

The writer is actually suggesting that for any internal medical problem more serious than pain control, it is better to go "underground" than to go to an MD. This is only one instance in which alternative medicine advocates seeking legitimacy are their own worst enemies.

The Web sites are full of fallacious claims and advice on the treatment of serious illnesses. The following example is not even an extreme case of Web site half-truths and misinformation. The Acupuncture.com site ran a news item under the headline "Alternative Medicine Popular for AIDS in Thailand." The item quoted *The Bangkok Post* as reporting that "the use of alternative medicine is the most effective therapy for patients with HIV/AIDS." If this were true, Thailand's financial crisis, as well as its AIDS epidemic, would be resolved. What the article was actually reporting was that there are 800,000 HIV-positive cases in Thailand. The cost of Western medicines, such as the antiretroviral drug AZT, is prohibitive in most situations there. Clinics and hospices have to use what they can afford, including Thai herbal medicine. The article went on to quote a hospice worker as saying that an herbal medicine called greater galangal (*Alpinia galanga* of the ginger family) is "very effective in treating patients with fungal problems in their mouth. Most HIV/AIDS patients have this mouth fungal problem and in my experience there is no modern medicine that is as effective as this herbal therapy" (<http://www.acupuncture.com/news/Thailand.html>).

This is a disturbing and misleading use of a news article to promote herbal medicine. The headline implies that alternative medicine is effective against AIDS. Actually it is just a report of Thai facilities that cannot afford modern drugs, pointing out the effectiveness of an herbal mouthwash. An herbal mouthwash is unlikely to cure HIV/AIDS. Once again the alternative medicine advocates are their own worst enemies. Misinformation such as this undermines the credibility of all reporting coming from the alternative health community, and prevents its relationship with the FDA and conventional medicine from developing beyond an adversarial position.

THE RCT STANDARD AND RECENT STUDIES

The litmus test or sterling standard of medical research held by both the AMA and the FDA is the RCCT (randomized controlled clinical test). The classic format is an experiment in which a sample group receives a drug or procedure being tested while a control group receives a placebo. Neither of the groups nor the medical personnel know who is receiving which treatment.

It is by such research results that drugs and treatments gain FDA approval and AMA endorsement. In 1998, the *Journal of the American Medical Association (JAMA)* devoted the November 11 issue to such studies of alternative medical research and discussion. In that *JAMA* issue and other AMA-affiliated publications, over eighty research articles and viewpoints were published. The *JAMA* editor stated that the purpose was to stem the "uncritical acceptance of untested and unproven alternative medical therapies" (Fontanarosa and Lundberg, 1998, p. 1619).

The research articles yielded a range of both positive and negative findings:

1. A study with pleasing results for the herbal community was published as "Treatment of Irritable Bowel Syndrome with Chinese Herbal Medicine." One difficulty in the previous scientific studies of TCM has been the issue of individualized diagnosis and dosage, in which the patient, not the disease, is treated. This Australian-based research recognized the importance, from the TCM perspective, of individualized treatment of patients even though they may all have the same medical problem. The researchers studied 116 patients diagnosed with irritable bowel syndrome (IBS). The study compared three treatments; an individualized TCM herbal therapy, a standardized TCM herbal formulation for IBS, "and a placebo using a randomized, double-blind, placebo-controlled study design" (Bensoussan et al., 1998, p. 1585).

Patients receiving the individualized herbal treatment and patients receiving the standardized herbal formula both responded significantly better than the placebo group. Interestingly, however, the patients receiving the individualized herbal treatment "had less improvement during treatment than patients receiving the standard formula, although this difference was not statistically significant" (Bensoussan et al., 1998, p. 1589).

Yet, like so much previous research done on Chinese herbal medicine, the results of this study were weakened since the study did not identify, by scientific name, the plants used, nor were the plant identities verified by any botanical authority. Furthermore, the specified dosage of five capsules, three times daily, is not meaningful without indicating the capsule size.

2. A currently popular herbal therapy was examined in "Saw Palmetto Extracts for Treatment of Benign Prostatic Hyperplasia." This study used the saw palmetto fruit extract, *Serenoa repens,* in prostate treatment. The results were quite positive in a "total of 18 randomized controlled studies involving 2,939 men." Compared to a commonly prescribed drug, finasteride, "*S. repens* produces similar improvement in urinary tract symptoms and urinary flow and was associated with fewer adverse treatment effects" (Wilt et al., 1998, p. 1604).

3. Yoga also showed promising results for a common, contemporary malady, in "Yoga-Based Intervention for Carpal Tunnel Syndrome." In "this preliminary study, a yoga-based regimen was more effective than wrist splinting or no treatment in relieving some symptoms and signs of carpal tunnel syndrome" (Garfinkel et al., 1998, p. 1601).

4. The chiropractic profession is least likely to applaud the results of a study of spinal manipulation in the treatment of tension-type headaches. The study concluded, "As an isolated intervention, spinal manipulation does not seem to have a positive effect on episodic tension-type headache" (Bove and Nilsson, 1998, p. 1576).

5. Due to its novelty and curiosity, the *JAMA* article on moxibustion was widely reported in U.S. newspapers. The study, "Moxibustion for Correction of Breech Presentation," was conducted in Jiangxi Province, People's Republic of China. Several newspapers reported findings to the effect that the ancient Chinese folk therapy had been demonstrated to be an effective preventive remedy for breech birth.

The article's more carefully worded conclusion was that among births diagnosed in late gestation as breech presentations, moxibustion treatment seemed to induce increased fetal activity and cephalic presentations (Cardini and Weixin, 1998, p. 1580).

Moxibustion is indeed an ancient medical practice in China and other Chinese-influenced cultures. It involves the burning of a compacted cigar-shaped stick of herbs very near the body's surface. The moxa burns flamelessly like a cigar, giving off heat, smoke, and a distinct odor. No authority is clear as to whether it is the heat or odor or smoke that is supposed to produce the efficacious result. Cardini reported that the primary herb used in her study was *Artemisia vulgaris* or mugwort. (As a personal comment, when I was treated in Nanning, Guangxi Autonomous Region, with moxibustion, the primary odor from the moxa was that of hemp. Though quite relaxing, I am unconvinced of its healing effect on my Bell's palsy at that time.)

In Cardini's study, the moxa was held at "acupoint BL 67 (Zhiyin) to promote version of fetuses in breech presentation . . . Acupoint BL 67 is beside the outer corner of the fifth toenail" (Cardini and Weixin, 1998, p. 1580). Cardini offers no theory or explanation of how it is that heat or smoke or odor stimulating the little toe produces this result, only suggesting that the method of moxibustion "is not entirely clear and warrants further research" (p. 1584).

Cardini also acknowledges that in regard to this study, "no randomized controlled trial has evaluated the efficacy of this therapy" (Cardini and Weixin, 1998, p. 1580).

Cardini further explains that the popularity of, and time-honored reliance upon, moxibustion for so many maladies in TCM creates a social atmosphere in which Cardini and Weixin felt it was "impossible to propose a 'sham moxibustion' that could serve as a control group; which is to say that the RCCT standard of medical research was culturally prohibited in this study. Additionally, Cardini acknowledges that in China moxibustion is a commonly "self-administered home therapy." The implication of this admission is that home-based moxibustion, outside of the control and knowledge of the researchers, could have been part of the data. This hardly meets the conditions of a controlled experiment (Cardini and Weixin, 1998, p. 1583).

Any reader attracted to acronyms will be tempted to say that the only real conclusion of this study is that you cannot do RCCT on TCM in the PRC. Even if one resists that indulgence, this study is still more ethnography than RCCT research. It illustrates the cultural resistance, or at least indifference, in China to proving or disproving the "science" of moxibustion specifically and TCM generally. Any scientific verification of the anecdotal efficacy of moxibustion or TCM will have to come from within the AMA-FDA cultural base. After all, it is only the AMA-FDA medical complex that is insisting on such proof. In this case, *JAMA* seems to be stretching its own standards to accommodate a culturally biased study.

This moxibustion study once again draws attention to the chasm separating the cultural history base of alternative research from the evidential base of scientific research.

The AMA, largely in reaction to the public's acceptance of alternative therapies, now seems committed to encouraging research that will establish a scientific basis for incorporating alternative therapies which meet its research standards. However, it will serve no purpose to publicize herbal medicine studies that are not scrupulous in validating the botanical species being used and in defining precisely the dosage forms and levels.

However, many alternative practitioners, for example acupuncturists and TCM dispensers, feel that such a scientific standard misses the point of holistic philosophy and denigrates or undermines their traditions and medical theories. Furthermore, they feel that the AMA intends to co-opt their therapies, thereby making alternative practitioners even more marginal to the medical world. Some alternative practitioners actually feel that their best interests lie, not in AMA acceptance and scientific respectability, but rather in emphasizing the nonevidential, "spiritual" or holistic base of their practice.

ACUPUNCTURE AND PLACEBO EFFECT

Acupuncture, especially, is in a catch-22 situation with regard to RCT research. Standard RCT research is based on comparing results between a group receiving acupuncture, a group receiving other pain therapy, and those receiving no therapy, or some such comparison. Results of such studies show positive results of acupuncture therapy for pain control and have gained NIH endorsement for specific pain relief uses. However, as reported by the NIH, the reasons acupuncture pain control can be effective remain unclear due to "inherent difficulties in the use of appropriate controls, such as placebos and sham acupuncture groups" (NIH Consensus Conference, 1998, p. 1518).

TCM theory cannot incorporate the concept of placebo effect. (How does a holistic theory distinguish an isolated aspect of treatment?) Therefore, all positive results, RCT or anecdotal, from a TCM perspective are proof of the efficacy of acupuncture. The catch-22 of holistic theory is that it cannot identify a single factor in treatment as being the causative factor. If a single factor is causative, then the explanation is no longer holistic. If the theory is holistic, the causation cannot be a single, isolated phenomenon.

This issue of placebo effect was crucial to the results in a *JAMA*-reported study of acupuncture treatments for HIV-related peripheral neuropathic pain, which concluded that acupuncture was not "more effective than placebo in relieving pain caused by HIV-related peripheral neuropathy" (Schlay et al., 1998, p. 1590).

The research team designed a "multicenter, modified double-blind, randomized, placebo-controlled study" of what they called "standardized acupuncture regimen" or SAR, involving 239 patients over fourteen weeks of SAR treatment (Schlay et al., 1998, p. 1590).

This study is a very good example of the inherent problems of scientifically studying acupuncture efficacy. First of all, to test the hypothesis of whether specific needling points promote analgesia, and to achieve a blinded and replicative design, the researchers administered *standardized* acupuncture for all patients. Classical TCM-based acupuncture requires individualized programs of acupuncture as diagnosed for each patient. "If the acupuncturists had used individualized treatment, the results would not be generalizable to other acupuncturists, and the treatment, if efficacious, could not have been used by other practitioners" (Schlay et al., 1998, pp. 1594-1595).

Here again is a catch-22 situation in which the rigors of scientific study require standardized conditions that can be replicated, while TCM theory requires individualized diagnosis and treatment. So if it's standardized, it isn't TCM; if it's individualistic, it's not science. Additionally there is the troubling question of whether the needling of "non-classical" or sham insertion points may have produced analgesic effects among the control group. How does an experimental researcher distinguish between real acupuncture points and sham points, or real acupuncture needle depth and sham depth (Margolin, Avants, and Kleber, 1998)?

The chasm between the two theoretical camps still remains. To satisfy scientific standards, acupuncture must be standardized and routinized. The acupuncture theorists will reject this as pseudoacupuncture. The researchers will reject anything less rigorous as pseudoscience.

The one clear certainty in this debate is that the stakes are rising in the long struggle over medicines and therapies in America. The cost of medical treatment of all varieties climbs each year. The billions of dollars ultimately involved nurtures this conflict more than it moves the protagonists toward resolution.

For all practical purposes, there now exists in the United States a de facto medical pluralism wherein millions of Americans are simultaneously seeing doctors and alternative therapists, or medicating themselves through dietary herbal supplements. In other words, too much medical care is as much a dilemma for many Americans as is too little for other segments of the population.

This situation means that each medical camp continues to judge the other by its own standards. The FDA-AMA view is that safe, effective therapies and products must be backed by costly long-term scientific study involving double-blind research. This view sees itself as protecting the health safety of the public.

The alternative medical view is that anecdotal evidence and the long history of use is proof enough, and that since small and midsized companies cannot afford to conduct long-term scientific research, only the huge international pharmaceutical companies will prevail if the law requires such research. This view presents itself as protecting the consumer choices and health freedoms of the public.

The establishment of a National Center for Complementary and Alternative Medicine, with a $50 million budget to fund research, will do virtually nothing to resolve this issue. Given the "true believer" nature of many American herbalists, the alternative/herbal community will agree with and laud any research validating their views, while rejecting any research results that do not confirm their faith. This is a typical response and a center for integral medicine will not affect this behavior.

As in so many areas of contemporary American life, honest and real differences in solutions to a sociological issue have hardened into ideological stances.

The AMA has at least moved from its previous "don't ask, don't tell" attitude toward patients using alternative therapies to a position in which doctors are encouraged to try to advise and monitor their patients' use of these therapies. However, the general response of self-appointed alternative spokespersons to this effort is defensive, fearing the co-optation of their functions by the AMA.

Meanwhile, Americans in search of health are voting with their checkbooks, spending comparable billions of dollars in the use of both medical models. American medicine users seem motivated by two attitudes: (1) a continuing faith in herbal/alternative practices despite widespread fraud and often only controversial proof of effectiveness; and (2) alienation and loss of faith in a medical system that is scientifically sound but increasingly impersonal, bureaucratic, and prone to arrogance. Such confused motives are almost certain to produce equally conflicted results.

Thus, fifty years after Dr. Cho's plea for communication between the two realms of medicine, both the consuming public and the health professionals are far from a level of interaction that would elevate medical care "like two wings of a bird."

Chapter 6

Placebos, Spontaneous Remissions, and Nonspecific Factors in Healing

The literal translation from Latin of the term placebo is "I shall please." The word itself was introduced into English usage in the fourteenth century as the popular name of a vespers sung for the dead and dying. This usage came from the Latin version of Psalm 116:9, "Placebo Domino in regione vivorum," usually translated as "I shall walk before the Lord in the land of the living." Over the years, the practice of administering a useless but harmless and soothing potion or herb came to be seen as the medical parallel to the singing of the vespers for the dying, and eventually shared the same name, placebo (Pepper, 1945).

Today the use of placebo and its effect is a widely acknowledged aspect of modern medical practice. Though there is an entire literature on the precise medical definition of placebo, it is usually agreed to be a nonspecific substance (substance having no specific curative effect) given to satisfy the psychophysiological needs of a patient, or as used on a control group in experimental design to further test the efficacy of an active substance or drug.

This would seem straightforward enough except that there is actually a wide range of disagreement among physicians, clinicians, psychiatrists, and philosophers of science as to just what constitutes a placebo and placebo effect (Grunbaum, 1989, p. 7).

In modern allopathic medicine, scientific medical care is virtually defined as "the therapeutic action of chemical substances" on biologically defined diseases and illnesses. This idea of "specific drugs for specific diseases" is a paramount and distinguishing feature of modern medicine (Shepherd and Sartorius, 1989, p. 1). And despite a grudging awareness of myriad contributing factors that influence treatment (physical-environmental, cultural, psychological), scientific medicine proceeds *as if* this were true.

Medical science acknowledges that physical, cultural, and psychological factors beyond the control of a physician affect the health of a patient. From a scientific view, the glory of a laboratory is that it is a controlled environment in which the influences of physical, cultural, and psychological factors are reduced as much as possible. An experiment is a process in which extreme effort is made to minimize these factors and to study, in splendid isolation, the therapeutic action of a designated substance. The goal of the efficient, antiseptic environment of the hospital is also to control and minimize the medically unintended consequences of the physical, cultural, psychological, outside world.

In modern medical parlance, all of these nonmedical elements that influence the health and treatment of a patient are called "nonspecific factors." The scientific medical goal is to isolate their influence to the degree that the specific and prescribed medical treatment can be proven effective. The attempt to do so may range from the simple instructions of when and how to take a prescribed drug to the stricter regimen of hospitalization or even quarantine. From a scientific perspective, modern medicine is constantly trying to insulate itself from the confusing and frustrating influences of placebo effects and nonspecific factors related to a patient's treatment.

It is generally acknowledged that psychotherapy is a field especially susceptible to nonspecific factors in treatment, and that many cases "where gains exceed those from spontaneous remission" may owe their improvement not to specific treatment or prescribed drugs, but "succeed for other reasons" which are largely unknown (Grunbaum, 1989, p. 8). Though not as candidly admitted, the same generalization applies to internal medicine as well.

The term mentioned in the previous paragraph, "spontaneous remission," is the third concept in what, from a scientific viewpoint, constitutes an unholy trinity, the other two parts of which are placebo and nonspecific factors.

Spontaneous remission describes the troubling persistence of a consistent percentage of diagnosed patients who show a marked and enduring improvement or complete disappearance of the diagnosed disease, for reasons that cannot be attributed to specific treatment. This holds true in virtually all diseases, including some forms of cancer (Lewison, 1976).

In other words, in a world where placebo, nonspecific factors, and spontaneous remission are real phenomena, even the most rigorously scientific medicine cannot account for a number of cases of marked improvement in the health or wellness of patients.

The attempt to comprehend and account for these subjective elements of medicine has led some scholars to endorse a broader definition of illness as "a social experience in the context of culture" (Eisenberg, 1983, p. 55). This sort of definition inevitably leads to the recognition that most of medical history in all societies has significantly been the history of placebos, nonspecific effects, and spontaneous remissions, with healers of various cultures and medical models taking credit whenever possible. Prior to the twentieth century in Western medicine, "doctors were largely engaged in the unwitting dispensation of placebos on a massive scale" (Shepherd and Sartorius, 1989, p. 8). Though Shepherd and Sartorius are writing specifically of the history of modern scientific medicine, this statement applies equally to alternative/herbal therapies, the difference being that scientific medicine now tries to distinguish between its drugs and placebo effects.

If it is misleading to describe pre-twentieth century medical treatment as "placebos on a massive scale," that is only because placebos are supposed to be harmless. Before physicians properly understood the concepts of antisepsis, contagion, and germ theory, a doctor's office or a hospital was surely the most likely place to contract a deadly illness. The time-honored practice of blood-letting probably killed as many as it "cured." As recently as the early 1900s, doctors "actually administered live hook-worms to patients with the disease, polycythemia, in which the body manufactures an excessive number of red blood cells" (Matthews and Clark, 1998, p. 179). In short, it seems no small achievement that the species has survived its medical history.

APPROACHING THERAPY

Throughout this study, the question of efficacy of treatment has stood like a wall separating scientific medicine from the alternative/herbal traditions. When presented with the question, "How does it work?" each camp rejects the answer of the other. Modern medicine rejects anecdotal and traditional proof. Alternative medicine rejects the necessity of scientific proof. Perhaps the useful question is not "How does it work?" but rather, "How does the patient best approach any therapy, alternative or conventional, in order to maximize the possibility of healing?"

Physicians as well as psychotherapists are acknowledging the role of the mind, or more precisely, the brain, in preparing the patient for healing. Herbert Benson, MD, is quoted as saying, "Our brains are wired for beliefs and expectancies. When activated the body can respond as it would if the belief were a reality" (Matthews and Clark, 1998, p. 178).

> Patients who believe that something is being done to control their illness and that they have a personal relationship with someone who will help them are less likely to be demoral-

ized and depressed. . . . Patients who are not demoralized and depressed are more likely to pay attention to personal hygiene, to eat and sleep better, to take medicine that has been prescribed, and to comply better with the therapist's other recommendations. All of these helpful behaviors will facilitate recovery. (Miller, 1989, p. 51)

APPROACHING PAIN

The human experience of pain, especially, seems to be one medical area where belief is tremendously powerful in shaping reality. Substantial research demonstrates the subjectivity of the experience of pain; that pain is influenced by placebo, by stress-induced analgesia, by anxiety, by behavioral conditioning, and by hypnosis (whatever hypnosis may be). Wartime studies show that a "good wound" that will get a soldier sent home is often experienced with low expression of pain. On the other hand, a traffic accident victim with less life-threatening injuries may typically express great pain and require sedation. Researchers theorize that the soldier may be exhibiting stress-induced analgesia, or the behavioral conditioning of military training; the accident victim's sufferings are linked to anxiety over insurance, hospitalization, loss of work, and so on. The point is that the experience of pain and its effect on the body can be highly influenced by the social setting and socioeconomic consequences of an injury (Miller, 1989, p. 49).

If pain can be influenced, then remediation of pain must have an equally strong subjective dimension. Certainly the nonspecific factors of the patient's perception of a particular drug therapy are well-documented. Children tend to expect more potency from large pills or capsules; adults usually associate very small tablets with great strength. Shape, color, and texture all influence the patient's perception of a drug. Multicolored capsules can be especially tricky; "one anxious patient reported that his minor tranquilizer worked better if he swallowed it green end first" (Joyce, 1989, p. 77). In the era of Prozac, Paxil, Xanax, Zantac, Zestril, and Zoloft, "it appears that pills must have the letter 'z' or 'x' in their names to be successful" (Matthews and Clark, 1998, p. 180). Perhaps all the flowers and references to nature on the packaging does improve the potency of herbal medicines.

An extreme example of the importance of patients' perceptions is a case of going to great pains for pain relief—the medical fad of angina pectoris surgery in the 1950s. In that era, many patients who reported the symptoms of angina pectoris, or heart pains, underwent internal mammary artery bypass surgery. Only after a "sham surgery" research study, in which one group of patients was given the bypass surgery and another group was simply cut open and then stitched up, was it determined that such surgery was not effective for angina pectoris. Results of the follow-up research showed that those undergoing the sham surgery were more likely to report "at least 50 per cent reduction in their angina pectoris (heart pain) one year later" (Matthews and Clark, 1998, p. 180). (Under today's standard of ethics on the use of human subjects in research, a study of this sort is no longer possible.)

FOUR FEATURES OF EFFECTIVE THERAPY

Dr. Jerome Frank has delineated what he considers to be the consistent features of effective psychotherapy: (1) an emotionally charged, confiding relationship with a helping person, often with the participation of a group; (2) a healing setting, which has at least two therapeutic functions in itself—it symbolizes the therapist's role as a healer and it provides safety; (3) a rationale, conceptual scheme, or myth that explains the patient's symptoms and prescribes a ritual or procedure for resolving them; and (4) a ritual that requires active participation of both patient and therapist (Frank, 1989, pp. 100-101).

Frank's four criteria offer a useful framework from which to again consider the question, "How does the patient best approach any therapy, alternative or conventional, to maximize the possibilities of healing?"

Emotional Relationship

Frank's first point focuses upon the patient's need for emotional support. No matter how physiologically based the ailment may be, whether broken leg, cut finger, or the like, people want some emotional sign of concern and care along with the cast or stitches. The more mysterious or internal the ailment, the greater is this need. Yet the very nature of a scientifically modeled medical relationship is that it is intended not to be emotionally charged. Doctors and their support staffs are trained to be emotionally distant in order to deal objectively with the cavalcade of sick and distraught who appear before them.

Objectivity, not subjectivity, is the acquired aura of conventional medical training. The white smocks, nurses' uniforms, and surgery scrubs may be functional, hygienic apparel, but they are also distancing costumes used to establish social space between the professional and the patient. These props are especially crucial for establishing social distance if the professional is going to explore the internal depths of the patient's body. Objectivity is wholly a state of mind while another human is probing your orifices.

The practice of internal medicine involves a physical intimacy between doctor and patient that in many ways rivals the intimacy between lovers. For that very reason, a doctor is trained in objectivity, to see a patient as an object or a set of symptoms. The degree of physical intimacy is supposed to be counterbalanced by an emotional distancing so that the relationship will be professional.

In regard to a confiding relationship, what modern doctor darting from cubicle to cubicle has time to listen? Patients spend more time in waiting rooms and then in examination rooms waiting for the doctor, than with the doctor.

In matters of emotional involvement and confiding, the very nature of the alternative models gives their practitioners the advantage. First of all, nearly all alternative models spend relatively more time interviewing the patient and compiling a case study. The focus on the person, rather than the disease, requires this sort of oral history. Because nearly all alternative models rely on natural and herbal therapies, the practitioner is less intrusive on the patient's body. Since the alternative professional is going to be less physically intimate, a greater degree of emotional intimacy is professionally acceptable. Furthermore, the alternative model's assumption of a physical-emotional-psychological unity, through which body and mind are reciprocally influential and capable of promoting self-healing, leads to the desirability of an emotionally supportive and confiding relationship conducive to healing.

In the area of "participation in a group," now even conventional practitioners of internal medicine are recognizing the utility of support groups comprising survivors and recovered patients. Alternative therapists also encourage this practice but also have a built-in support group system in the form of alternative medicine's transmission through the years by the anecdotal testimony of previous patients.

Throughout these pages, the point has been reiterated that, from the scientific perspective, alternative medicine's reliance on anecdotal proof is an inherent systemic weakness. However, that weakness is also a strength in the sense that the collective body of anecdotal testimony from past and current users of alternative therapies constitutes a shared belief system. It comes from a community of believers whom the patient is invited to join by also being healed or cured via alternative medicine. The alternative medicine Web sites and chat rooms are, in this sense, medical versions of radio-television evangelism, to which the sick can always "log on." These media-based anecdotes and testimonies of healing, along with a patient's personal associations, create an extensive support system, reaching through space and back in time; and it is far more accessible and emotionally comforting to the average person than is the scientific objectivity and research base of conventional medicine.

A Healing Setting, Symbolizing the Therapist's Role As a Healer and Providing Safety

The physical setting of the healing process has changed radically in the lifetime and experience of America's older patients. Who among us can remember seeing the doctor in his or her office? Today, it is a distinctly old-fashioned practice wherein the doctor sitting at a desk greets a patient, discusses symptoms, and moves the patient about the office to scales, examining stool, examination table, and so on. The great disadvantage of this old office format was that the doctor presiding in the office could see only one patient at a time. Though this arrangement might give the patient a comforting sense of full attention, it was financially disadvantageous to the business aspect of the medical practice. Surely, somewhere in a 1950s issue of *Medical Economics,* there is a full rationale (with floor plan) for the reorganization of the healing setting into its present form.

The contemporary medical setting of a series of examination cubicles allows the doctor to scurry from patient to patient, examining the tonsils of one while another is undressing and putting on a paper gown. And though the doctor may have photocopies of certificates and diplomas, affirming his or her healing qualifications, on a wall of each cubicle, these still leave the patient with long moments in a literally sterile environment.

So far as conveying a sense of safety, these little rooms are safe enough in the same sense that an OSHA-inspected workplace is relatively accident-proof. Also, you know that you are insured; otherwise you would not be there.

Without insurance, your medical experiences will be restricted to ER facilities. There, due to crowding, you will be triaged in terms of the immediacy of your need for attention. While waiting, your idea of good fortune swings perversely. If lucky enough to have only a minor ailment or injury, you will have a long wait during which to count your blessings. After a few hours, you may begin to wish you had a gushing wound like those ushered in ahead of you. If surgery should be required, you will be given a waiver to sign, thereby heading off any nuisance lawsuits against the healing setting. (There must somewhere exist research showing that the signing of such waiver forms counteracts any potential placebo effect and is therefore counterproductive to treatment.)

Overall, in most persons' experience, the various symbols of the business setting are a powerful antidote undermining the symbols of the healing setting. The insurance forms, liability forms, and waiver forms suggest that the safety of the medical business weighs as heavily in importance as the safety of the sick. Though this may not be true, the perception remains. In any discussion of the symbols of healing and safety, perception is important.

A Conceptual Rationale or Myth That Explains the Patient's Symptoms and Prescribes a Ritual or Procedure for Resolving Them

Dr. Frank is using the term "myth" in the sense of a theory that offers understanding, and "ritual" as action or conduct that supports the myth. "By inspiring expectations of help, myths and rituals not only help keep the patient coming to treatment, but may also be powerful morale builders and symptom relievers in themselves." Research also suggests that expectations of help are further supported if "hope for improvement" is "linked in the patient's mind to a specific process of therapy" (Frank, 1989, pp. 101-102).

A Ritual That Requires Active Participation of Both Patient and Therapist

Doctors of conventional medicine often assume that their patients are already familiar with and confident of the therapies and medications being offered. Thus, they spend less time in aiding or instructing the patient toward associating hope for improvement with a particular therapy.

Practitioners of alternative therapies generally assume that their patients need direction in becoming familiar and confident with an alternative treatment. They tend to spend relatively more time in initial sessions instructing and building the patient's confidence in the procedure. They want the patient to assume "ownership" of the process. "Introducers of new or unfamiliar therapies regularly spend considerable time and effort at the start teaching the patient their particular therapeutic game and shaping the patient's expectations accordingly." A body of research points to "a consistent, modestly positive relationship between patient preparation and patient improvement" (Frank, 1989, pp. 102-103). The arousal of hope seems to be transformed into the expectation of help.

So by their conduct and procedures, the practitioners of alternative therapies tend to offer more actively involving myth and ritual than do conventional doctors. Probably by self-selection, persons more comfortable with such concepts as myth and ritual have gravitated to the various alternative medical fields. Here, especially, the practitioners of TCM and other Asian-based models may have a distinct strength in their association with the exotic symbolism and paraphernalia of Asian traditions.

In terms of placebo effect, nonspecific aspects of treatment, and spontaneous remission, all that any myth and ritual may do is to create in the patient's mind the conditions of maximum receptivity to the possibilities of the three processes.

A patient under the guidance of such a therapist has the advantage of being urged along in a healing myth and ritual. But what about the millions of people whose primary experience of alternative medicines is the dietary supplements that they consume, essentially without medical guidance? A great many people taking these items are self-medicating on the basis of self-diagnosis. Putting aside for the moment the real dangers of wrong medication and overmedication, the people who are self-diagnosed and self-medicated are involved in a personal myth of self-knowledge.

However misguided, the level of self-interest needed to follow a regimen of self-medication may constitute an involving, responsibility-centered myth and ritual equal in effect to one directed by a therapist. Herbal medicines, especially, with their low-potency, long-term dosages, require long-term self-monitoring and self-awareness; during which the lifestyle of medication, proper diet, and adequate rest may be as efficacious as most supervised therapy. It would be intriguing to speculate on just how much healing could be attributed to the nonspecific influences of such a behavior pattern, rather than the herbal potions themselves.

Earlier in the text, the unifying themes of alternative medicines were listed:

1. A physical-spiritual-psychological unity through which body and mind are reciprocally influential, and capable of promoting self-healing
2. Natural therapies and herbs being considered preferable to medical technologies and drugs
3. The importance of diet and nutrition, based on herbs and whole foods, to health

In the sense that the term "myth" is being discussed, these three themes outline the myth of alternative medicine. Its great advantage over the myth of scientific medicine is that it is extremely inclusive and involving. The rigors of the scientific method require conventional medicine to be obsessive in excluding all methods, results, and nonspecific aspects of treatment that are not statistically verifiable. That is the lonely beauty of science; but by its nature, it is not very involving or accessible to the average person or patient.

The very language of conventional medicine distances the patient from its myth. Conventional medicine speaks of surgery that corrects the malfunctioning organ, procedures that clear the arteries, chemicals that destroy the cancerous cells, or antibacterials that kill the infection. The drugs or procedures or chemicals are described as the active participants, while the patient is the field upon which the action takes place. There is an undeniable majesty to scientific medicine, but it is not successful in providing its patients with an involving myth and ritual.

Conversely, alternative medicine speaks of the unity of body, soul, and mind. It stresses that illness is defeated through self-healing, in which the patient is an active participant. It emphasizes that health is a harmonic relationship between persons and surroundings; that a diet and lifestyle rooted in nature is the key to wellness. Yet, alternative medicine's greatest asset may be that its myth has absorbed and included placebo effect, nonspecific influences, and spontaneous remission as integral elements of the process of herbal/natural healing. Quite unintentionally, and long before those terms were in use, TCM, Ayurvedic medicine, naturopathy, herbal healing, and so on, all subsumed this trinity, not distinguishing between these processes and the prescribed therapy, but rather assuming that a therapy which maximizes the potentiality of healing would include these three processes.

Having co-opted placebo, nonspecific influences, and spontaneous remission into its inclusive myth of healing, alternative medicine may, with logical consistency, simply include their positive effects as part of its healing efficacy and reported cures. For this reason, if no other, alternative medicine will continue to be perceived as useful and will grow in use in any foreseeable future of medicine.

Chapter 7

Herbal Medicine:
The German Example

In the past, but also continuing today, many different schools of herbalists have operated from a romantic perspective that the healing power of herbal treatment derives from a spiritual-holistic base, that some ritual process is crucial to the healing, and that some special esoteric knowledge or communion with nature is at the source of wellness. These vestiges of a shamanistic perspective, regardless of their efficacy, are a major barrier preventing large-scale incorporation of herbal medicines into scientific, mainstream medical practice.

In the previous chapter, the placebo power of ritual and emotional support, at which many traditional herbalists excel, was discussed in terms of its healing utility. But for the moment, putting aside these real and valuable elements of treatment, some pragmatic questions remain: (1) Do traditional herbalists really know the epidemiology of what they are treating? (2) Are their prescriptive skills based on a sure knowledge of the plant materials they use? (3) Will the crude plant materials used by traditional herbalists yield the qualitative and quantitative dosage of active ingredient that will ameliorate the medical problem?

The first two questions are endlessly controversial, and have been debated for decades by the opposing camps. There is a point at which pursuing these tradition-versus-science issues is counterproductive. However, the third question is now more likely to yield an answer based on evidence rather than opinion. The focus on this question is part of the development of what some experts have called "rational phytotherapy." Rational phytotherapy's distinctive feature is the standardization of herb- and plant-based medicines. It has developed from the realization that herbs can have medical efficacy, but only through the standardization of qualitative and quantitative dosage.

> Herbs are natural products. Nature does not supply its products with a consistent, standardized composition . . . the constituents of medical herbs can vary greatly as a result of genetic factors, climate, soil quality, and other external factors. The material derived from cultivated medicinal plants shows smaller variations than material gathered from the wild. . . . Thus, standardization of the extract begins with selection and mixing of the herbal raw materials. (Schulz, Hänsel, and Tyler, 1998, p. 6)*

If nothing else, this should at least lay to rest the issue of wild versus cultivated herbs. Cultivated herbs are a more reliable source of medicine than those found in the wild.

Following the pattern of the use and acceptance of rational phytotherapy in Europe, and especially Germany, the future of herbal medicine will more closely resemble the modern pharmaceutical industry than the village herbalist.

> Phytomedicines are medicinal plants that contain plant materials as their pharmacologically active component. . . . For most phytomedicines, the specific ingredients that determine the pharmacologic activity are unknown. The crude drug (dried herb) or a whole extract derived from it is considered to be the active ingredient. (Schulz, Hänsel, and Tyler, 1998, p. 4)

---

*All quotes from Schulz, V., R. Hänsel, and V. Tyler, *Rational Phytotherapy,* Third Edition, copyright © 1998, reprinted with permission from Springer-Verlag, Berlin.

The key word distinguishing phytotherapy from traditional herbalism is "extracts," which "are concentrated preparations of a liquid, powdered, or viscous consistency that are ordinarily made from dried plant parts (the crude drug) by maceration or percolation. . . . Two key factors determine the internal composition of an extract: the quality of the herbal raw material and the production process" (Schulz, Hänsel, and Tyler, 1998, pp. 5-6).

Even laboratory-produced plant extracts are sometimes of dubious quality due to the raw materials used. Commercial producers operate in a marketplace where brokers and suppliers offer surplus and ungraded raw materials at cut-rate prices. The PharmaPrint report of inferior ginseng is only one instance of poor quality herbs sold for medicinal processing. PharmaPrint's decision to report this was more unusual than the transaction itself.

Advocates of phytotherapy point to Germany as having the most enlightened standards, controls, and legislation:

In Germany, the use of plant drugs is a science . . . the principal reason is, without question, the enlightened system of laws and regulations governing the sale and use of such products in that country.

Basically, the regulations in Germany permit phytomedicines to be sold either as self-selected or prescription drugs provided there is absolute proof of their safety and reasonable certainty of the efficacy. The words "reasonable certainty" are extremely important here. They require that some scientific and clinical evidence be provided prior to approval, but the requirements are not the same as would be necessary for a new chemical entity. Because patent protection it [*sic*] not ordinarily available for these ancient drugs, pharmaceutical companies are generally unwilling to invest the hundreds of millions of dollars required to prove them effective by the same standards applied to totally new synthetic drugs. They are, however, willing to invest more modest amounts in the scientific and clinical testing needed to establish reasonable certainty of efficacy.

That has been and continues to be done in Germany. Data regarding safety and efficacy submitted to a specific body designated Commission E of the German Federal Health Agency (now the Federal Institute for Drugs and Medical Devices) have resulted in judgments validating the utility of several hundred different phytomedicines. (Schulz, Hänsel, and Tyler, 1998, pp. v-vi)

The most frequently approved phytotherapies in Germany are those classified as single-herb products:

In 1995, phytomedicines accounted for approximately 7 percent of all prescription medications covered by public health insurance in Germany, with total sales of about 2 billion DM. Two-thirds of the prescriptions were for single-herb products, i.e., products whose active ingredients derive from only one medicinal plant. Just 5 herbs account for approximately 60 percent of these prescriptions, and 28 herbs account for more than 90 percent. (Schulz, Hänsel, and Tyler, 1998, p. ix)

Among the most commonly prescribed herbal medications in Germany, the best selling single-herb product is ginkgo biloba, followed by St. John's wort. Ginkgo biloba has been used in TCM for centuries. Today its primary TCM use is in treating asthma. Western research has placed ginkgo extract among "the class of nootropic drugs, i.e., agents that act on the central nervous system and tend to improve cognitive performance" (Schulz, Hänsel, and Tyler, 1998, p. 43).

China and other east Asian areas, as well as France and the United States, continue to be the primary sources of the bulk plant materials. The leaves of the plant yield the desired extract, high in flavonoid glycosides. The extract content is influenced by the time of harvest and condition of tree, as well as soil and climate.

In Germany, only the extracts (not the leaves themselves) meeting strict standards can be used in herbal medicines for human use. The standardized extraction "process eliminates unwanted components, including those that make the product less stable or pose an excessive toxocologic risk—fats, waxes, tannins, proanthocyanidins, biflavonoids, ginkgol, ginkgolic acids, proteins, and mineral components. The extracts suitable for use in drug manufacture are designated in the technical literature as EGb 761 and LI 1370" (Schulz, Hänsel, and Tyler, 1998, p. 40).

A substantial body of research literature on the pharmacologic efficacy of ginkgo biloba extract-based drugs has been published in Germany, meeting the standards of the German government. "The *Rote Liste 1995* (Red List—the German equivalent of *Physician's Desk Reference*) contains a total of eight allopathic ginkgo preparations, five of which meet the specifications of the 1994 Commission E monograph (extracts EGb 761 and LI 1370); the three others do not" (Schulz, Hänsel, and Tyler, 1998, p. 48).

St. John's wort and all other single-herb phytotherapies, are held to the same high standard in Germany. St. John's wort (*Hypericum perforatum*) has been used for centuries in Europe and Asia for mood disorders. As an herbal antidepressant, it is now one of the most widely used herbal medicines in the world (which may also say something about the current mood in the world). The plant grows throughout Europe, Asia, and North and South America. Solid clinical evidence confirms the efficacy of St. John's wort extract-based preparations "in the treatment of depression or at least certain of its symptoms. . . . The *Rote Liste 1995* identifies 18 single-herb hypericum products that are marketed in Germany" (Schulz, Hänsel, and Tyler, 1998, pp. 60, 63).

The distinction between rational phytotherapies (plant-based drugs for which safety has been scientifically documented) and other herbal remedies has increased the medical choices of German consumers and given them a prescription option that is usually less costly than conventional drugs. German drug law has laid the basis for this expansion of choices.

> The fifth amendment of the German Drug Law of August 9, 1994, laid the groundwork for drawing a distinction between rational and irrational plant medicines. This amendment states that scientifically proven phytomedicines (most likely single-herb products) will be evaluated for pharmaceutical quality, efficacy, and safety in a normal approval process and will be given a corresponding approval number that physicians can recognize. (Schulz, Hänsel, and Tyler, 1998, pp. 14-15)

This German experience seems to be an excellent example of how scientific allopathic medicine can incorporate hundreds of herbal therapies without compromising scientific standards. The relevant question is whether this path could be taken in the United States. If, as the *JAMA* editor stated in the November 11, 1998 issue, the AMA goal is to halt the "uncritical acceptance of untested and unproven alternative medical therapies," then emulating the German example of the promotion of rational phytotherapy would seem to be a very good starting point.

The research base is available. If the AMA does not choose to accept the existing studies, then, as with all real science, these studies can be replicated. Any such solution, in reality, would have to be implemented through the coordinated effort of the FDA, NIH, AMA, and the pharmaceutical industry. This medical-industrial complex of government regulation, research efforts, professional standards, and industrial wealth is the power base from which all medical change in America is instigated. For the time being, at least, the AMA is showing signs of wanting to respond to the growing use of alternative medicine in America. Their stated concern is the indiscriminate nature of this use. Urging the FDA and pharmaceutical companies to examine rational phytotherapy would be an excellent first step toward minimizing the nonrational medical decisions now being made by so many patients.

This suggestion assumes that the users of alternative medicine are looking for rational medicine. The previous chapter emphasizes the human penchant for myth, ritual, and a holistic/spiritual explanation of healing. In the face of any rational therapy, some alternative medicine users are certain to stick to their romantic inclinations.

This suggestion also ignores the very likely resistance of some dietary supplement companies to such changes. Despite their vilification of the FDA, many dietary supplement manufacturers have successfully adapted to the FDA designation of their goods as food products, not drugs. A transition to rational phytotherapy in the United States would necessitate significant research expenditures by the dietary supplement manufacturers and thrust them into direct competition with the large pharmaceutical companies.

Throughout these chapters, there have been examples of the conflict between the rational and the subjective:

- The continued preference for "wild" herbs when scientific evidence shows cultivated herbs to be more uniform and at least equally efficacious
- The slaughter of bears in the absence of evidence of the efficacy of bear bile potions
- The continued fantasy world of aphrodisiacs in the age of Viagra
- The elusive Qi of TCM
- The absence of explanation for how acupuncture or moxibustion work

Irrationality will persist in medical choice and practice. Even as the paragon of scientific medicine, the AMA, still cherishes its caduceus as a symbol of its traditional origins, so do its patients expect physicians to maintain some link to the realm of the human spirit in their practice. Physicians who lose that link run the risk of losing their patients to alternative practitioners, some of whom offer little else. Medical pluralism is now as much a part of American medicine as it is a part of the medicine of developing nations.

Bibliography

Print Sources

Achord, J.L. Is Oriental use of bear bile vindicated (yet)? *Gastroenterology* 98, 1990, 1090-1991.

Ashland Daily Tidings. Researchers say echinacea has little effect on common cold. November 12, 1998, 6.

Bensky, D. and A. Gamble. *Chinese Herbal Medicine: Materia Medica.* Seattle, WA: Eastland Press. 1986.

Bensoussan, A., N.J. Talley, M. Hing, R. Menzies, A. Guo, and M. Ngu. Treatment of irritable bowel syndrome with Chinese herbal medicine. *Journal of the American Medical Association.* November 11, 1998, 280(18): 1585-1589.

Bertschinger, R. Medical texts in China. In *Encyclopaedia of the History of Science, Technology, and Medicine in Non-Western Cultures*, H. Selin (Ed.), pp. 673-676. Dordrecht, The Netherlands: Kluwer Academic Publishers. 1997.

Blass, A. East cures West. *Far East Economic Review.* October 21, 1993, 36-38.

Bove, G. and N. Nilsson. Spinal manipulation in the treatment of episodic tension-type headache. *Journal of the American Medical Association.* November 11, 1998, 280(18): 1576-1579.

Brevort, P. The booming U.S. botanical market. *HerbalGram.* No. 44, 1998, 33-46.

Burghart, R. Penicillin: An ancient Ayurvedic medicine. In *The Context of Medicines in Developing Countries*, S. Van Der Geest and S.R. Whyte (Eds.), pp. 289-298. Dordrecht, The Netherlands: Kluwer Academic Publishers. 1988.

Burros, M. A little medicine with your food. *The New York Times.* December 30, 1998, B12.

Cai, Jingfeng. Medicine in China. In *Encyclopaedia of the History of Science, Technology, and Medicine in Non-Western Cultures*, Dordrecht, The Netherlands: Kluwer Academic Publishers. 1997.

Capasso, L. 5300 years ago, the Ice Man used natural laxatives and antibiotics. *The Lancet.* December 5, 1998, 1864.

Cardini, F. and Weixin, H. Moxibustion for correction of breech presentation. *Journal of the American Medical Association.* November 11, 1998, 280(18): 1580-1584.

Castleman, M. Ginseng revered and reviled. *Herb Quarterly.* No. 48, Winter 1990, 17-24.

Cho, H.Y. *Oriental Medicine: A Modern Interpretation.* K. Kim, Trans. Compton, CA: Yuin University Press. 1996.

Complimentary and Alternative Medicine at the NIH (newsletter). Washington, DC: Office of Alternative Medicine Clearing House. 5(2), Spring 1998.

Consumer Reports. Herbal roulette. November 1995, 698-705.

Cui, J., M. Garle, P. Eneroth, and I. Bjorkhem. What do commercial ginseng preparations contain? *The Lancet.* 344, July 9, 1994, 134.

Desai, P.N. Medical ethics in India. In *Encyclopaedia of the History of Science, Technology, and Medicine in Non-Western Cultures.* H. Selin (Ed.), pp. 669-671. Dordrecht, The Netherlands: Kluwer Academic Publishers. 1997.

Eisenberg, D.M., R.C. Kessler, C. Foster, F.E. Norlock, D.R. Calkins, and T.L. Delbanco. Unconventional medicine in the United States. *New England Journal of Medicine.* January 28, 1993, 246-252.

Eisenberg, L. The subjective in medicine. *Perspectives in Biology and Medicine.* 27(1), 1983, 48-61.

Espinoza, E., J.A. Shafer, and L.R. Hagey. International trade in bear gallbladders: Forensic source inference. *Journal of Forensic Sciences.* No. 6, November 1993, 1363-1371.

Farve, D.S. *International Trade in Endangered Species: A Guide to CITES.* Norwell, MA: Martinus Nijhoff Publishers. 1989.

Farve, D.S. *Wildlife Law.* Charlotte, MI: Lupus Publishers. 1991.

Fitzgerald, S. *Whose Business Is It?* Washington, DC: World Wildlife Fund. 1989.

Fontanarosa, P.B. and G.D. Lundberg. Alternative medicine meets science. *Journal of the American Medical Association.* November 11, 1998, 280(18): 1618-1619.

Forestier-Walker, K. Hong Kong tests Chinese medicine. *New Scientist.* No. 1585, 1987, 47-50.

Foster, S. and Yue Chongxi. *Herbal Emissaries Bring Chinese Herbs to the West.* Rochester, VT: Healing Arts Press. 1992.

Foster, S. and V.E. Tyler. *Tyler's Honest Herbal,* Fourth Edition. Binghamton, NY: The Haworth Press. 1999.

Frank, J.D. Non-specific aspects of treatment: The view of a psychotherapist. In *Non-Specific Aspects of Treatment.* M. Shepherd and N. Sartorius (Eds.), pp. 95-114. Toronto: Hans Huber Publishers. 1989.

Fu Li-kuo (Ed. in Chief). *China Plant Red Data Book,* Vol. I. Beijing: Science Press. 1992.

Fuller, D. *Medicine from the Wild.* Washington, DC: World Wildlife Fund. 1991.

Garfinkel, M.S., A. Singhal, W.A. Katz, D.A. Allan, R. Reshetar, and R. Schumacher. Yoga-based intervention for carpal tunnel syndrome. *Journal of the American Medical Association.* November 11, 1998, 280(18): 1601-1603.

Gaski, A.L. and K.A. Johnson. *Prescription for Extinction: Endangered Species and Patented Oriental Medicines in Trade.* Washington, DC: World Wildlife Fund. 1994.

Golden, T. About heart in San Francisco. *Detroit Free Press.* August 27, 1996, 5A.

Greimel, H. Oregon authorities using racketeering laws against poachers. *The Ashland Daily Tidings.* September 26, 1998, 5.

Grunbaum, A. The placebo concept in medicine and psychiatry. In *Non-Specific Aspects of Treatment*. M. Shepherd and N. Sartorius (Eds.), pp. 7-38. Toronto: Hans Huber Publishers. 1989.

Hagey, L.R., D.L. Crombie, E. Espinosa, M. Carey, H. Igimi, and A.F. Hofmann. Ursodeoxychycholic acid in the Ursidae: Biliary bile acids of bears, pandas, and related carnivores. *Journal of Lipid Research*. 34, 1993, 1911-1916.

Hainer, C. Healing's lost horizons. *USA Today*. September 18, 1998, 5D.

Harding, A.R. *Ginseng and Other Medicinal Plants*. Boston, MA: Emporium Publications. 1972. (Originally published 1908.)

Hemley, G. *International Wildlife Trade: A CITES Sourcebook*. Washington, DC: World Wildlife Fund. 1994.

Hube, K. More insurers pick up the tab for alternative medicine. *Money Magazine*. October 1996, 25.

Inskipp, T. *World Checklist of Threatened Mammals*. Cambridge, UK: World Conservation Monitoring Centre. 1993.

Japsen, B. FDA could supplement vitamin regulation. *Chicago Tribune*. September 6, 1998, section 1, 1, 19.

Joyce, C.R.B. Non-specific aspects of treatment from the point of view of a clinical pharmacologist. In *Non-Specific Aspects of Treatment*. M. Shepherd and N. Sartorius (Eds.), pp. 57-94. Toronto: Hans Huber Publishers. 1989.

Ko, R.J. Adulterants in Asian patent medicines. *The New England Journal of Medicine*. September 17, 1998, 847.

La Pierre, Y. Illicit harvest. *National Parks Magazine*. May-June 1994, 33-37.

Lee, R.P.L. Perceptions and uses of Chinese medicine among the Chinese in Hong Kong. *Culture, Medicine, and Psychiatry*, No. 4, 1980, 345-375.

Leslie, C. (Ed.). *Asian Medical Systems*. Berkeley, CA: University of California Press. 1976.

Leslie, C. and A. Young. *Paths to Asian Medical Knowledge*. Delhi: Munshiram Manoharlal Publishers. 1933.

Lewison, E.F. (Ed.). *Conference on Spontaneous Remission of Cancer*. National Cancer Institute Monograph 44. Bethesda, MD: U.S. Dept. of Health, Education, and Welfare. 1976.

Lovelock, J.E. *The Ages of Gaia: A Biography of Our Living Earth*. New York: Norton Publishers. 1988.

Margolin, A., S.K. Avants, and H.D. Kleber. Investigating alternative medicine therapies in randomized control trials. *Journal of the American Medical Association*. November 11, 1998, 280(18): 1626-1628.

Marwick, C. Alterations are ahead at the OAM. *Journal of the American Medical Association*. November 11, 1998, 280(18): 1553-1554.

Matthews, D.A. and C. Clark. *The Faith Factor*. New York: Viking Press. 1998.

McCracken, C.D., A. Rose, and K.A. Johnson. *Status, Management, and Commercialization of the American Black Bear (Ursus Americanus)*. Seattle, WA: Eastland Press. 1986.

Miller, N.E. Placebo factors in treatment: Views of a psychologist. In *Non-Specific Aspects of Treatment*. M. Shepherd and N. Sartorius (Eds.), pp. 39-55. Toronto: Hans Huber Publishers. 1989.

Mills, J. Milking the bear trade. *International Wildlife*. May/June 1992, 38-45.

Mills, J.A. and C. Servheen. *The Asian Trade in Bears and Bear Parts*. Washington, DC: World Wildlife Fund. 1991.

NIH Consensus Conference, Panel on Acupuncture. Acupuncture. *Journal of the American Medical Association*. November 4, 1998, 280(17): 1518-1524.

Nowell, K., Chyi Wei Lein, and P. Chica-jai. *The Horns of a Dilemma*. London: World Wildlife Fund. 1992.

Ohnuki-Tierney, E. *Illness and Culture in Contemporary Japan*. New York: Cambridge University Press. 1984.

Pepper, O.H.P. A note on the placebo. *American Journal of Pharmacy*. 117, 1945, 409-412.

Reid, D.P. *Chinese Herbal Medicine*. Boston, MA: Shambala Press. 1993.

Schlay, J.C., K. Chaloner, M.B. Max, B. Flaws, P. Reichelderfer, D. Wentworth, S. Hillman, B. Brizz, and D.L. Cohn. Acupuncture and amitriptyline for pain due to HIV-related peripheral neuropathy. *Journal of the American Medical Association*. November 11, 1998, 280(18): 1590-1595.

Schulz, V., R. Hänsel, and V.E. Tyler. *Rational Phytotherapy*. Third Edition. Berlin: Springer-Verlag. 1998.

Sheldrake, R. *The Rebirth of Nature*. Rochester, VT: Destiny Books. 1994.

Shepherd, M. and N. Sartorius (Eds.). *Non-Specific Aspects of Treatment*. Toronto: Hans Huber Publishers. 1989.

Siegel, R.K. Ginseng abuse syndrome: Problems with the panacea. *Journal of the American Medical Association*. 1979, 241(15): 1614-1615.

Slifman, N.R., W.R. Obermeyer, B.K. Aloi, S.M. Musser, W.A. Correll, S.M. Cichowicz, J. Betz, and L.A. Love. Contamination of botanical dietary supplements by *Digitalis Lanata*. *The New England Journal of Medicine*. September 17, 1998, 806-811.

Strohecker, J. *Alternative Medicine: The Definitive Guide*. Puyallup, WA: Future Medicine Publishing, Inc. 1994.

Unschuld, P.U. Culture and pharmaceutics: Some epistemological observations of pharmacological systems in ancient Europe and medieval China. In *The Context of Medicines in Developing Countries*. S. Van Der Geest and S.R. Whyte (Eds.), pp. 179-197. Dordrecht, The Netherlands: Kluwer Academic Publishers. 1988.

Wesdock, J. Black pearl—A Chinese herbal remedy as an explanation for a positive urine drug test for oxazopam. *MRO Update*. April, 1998, 7-8.

Wilkinson, J. The signature of plants. *Kindred Spirits*. 1997, 3(4): 36-38.

Wilt, T.J., A. Ishani, G. Stark, R. MacDonald, J. Lau, and C. Mulrow. Saw palmetto extracts for treatment of benign prostatic hyperplasia. *Journal of the American Medical Association*. November 11, 1998, 280(18): 1604-1609.

Internet Sources

Acupuncture.com, <http://www.acupuncture.com>
Alternative Health Insurance, <http://www.alternative-insurance.com>
Bear Watch, <http://www.bearwatch.org>
Family and Fitness, <http://www.familyandfitness.com>
Fast.quote.com, <http://www.fast.quote.com>
Import Alert #6610, <http://www.fda.gov/ora/fiars/ora_import_ia6610.html>
International Advocates for Health Freedom, <http://www.iahf.com>
Life Extension Foundation, <http://www.lef.org>
Market Place, <http://cbc.ca/consumers/market/files/health/herbdrugs.html>
Medwatch, <http://www.pharminfo.com/medwatch/mwrpt36.html>
Message from Jackie Chan, <http://www.jackiewild.com>
Natural HealthLine, <http://www.naturalhealthvillage.com>
Picker Institute, <http://www.picker.com>
U.S. Fish and Wildlife Service, <http://www.fws.gov/r9dia/asian/html>
Viable Herbal Solutions, <http://www.lef.org>

Index

THE HAWORTH HERBAL PRESS
Varro E. Tyler, PhD
Executive Editor

UNDERSTANDING ALTERNATIVE MEDICINE: NEW HEALTH PATHS IN AMERICA by Lawrence Tyler. (2000). "An insightful view into several aspects of the alternative therapy movement that are often overlooked." *Karen Horneffer, PhD, Holistic Health Care Program, Western Michigan University, Kalamazoo, MI*

SEASONING SAVVY: HOW TO COOK WITH HERBS, SPICES, AND OTHER FLAVORINGS by Alice Arndt. (1999). "Well-written and wonderfully comprehensive exploration of the world of herbs, spices, and aromatics—at once authoritative and easy to use." *Nancy Harmon Jenkins, Author of* The Mediterranean Diet Cookbook

TYLER'S HONEST HERBAL: A SENSIBLE GUIDE TO THE USE OF HERBS AND RELATED REMEDIES, Fourth Edition by Steven Foster and Varro E. Tyler. (1999). "An up-to-date revision of the most reliable source for the layperson on herbal medicines. Excellent as a starting point for scientists who desire more information on herbal medicines." *Norman R. Farnsworth, PhD, Research Professor of Pharmacognosy, College of Pharmacy, University of Illinois at Chicago*

TYLER'S HERBS OF CHOICE: THE THERAPEUTIC USE OF PHYTOMEDICINALS, Second Edition by James E. Robbers and Varro E. Tyler. (1999). "The first edition of this book was a landmark publication. . . . This new edition will no doubt become one of the most often-used references by health practitioners of all types." *Mark Blumenthal, Founder and Executive Director, American Botanical Council; Editor,* Herbalgram

Order Your Own Copy of
This Important Book for Your Personal Library!

UNDERSTANDING ALTERNATIVE MEDICINE
New Health Paths in America

_____ in hardbound at $49.95 (ISBN: 0-7890-0741-X)

_____ in softbound at $19.95 (ISBN: 0-7890-0902-1)

COST OF BOOKS_____

OUTSIDE USA/CANADA/
MEXICO: ADD 20%_____

POSTAGE & HANDLING_____
*(US: $3.00 for first book & $1.25
for each additional book)
Outside US: $4.75 for first book
& $1.75 for each additional book)*

SUBTOTAL_____

IN CANADA: ADD 7% GST_____

STATE TAX_____
*(NY, OH & MN residents, please
add appropriate local sales tax)*

FINAL TOTAL_____
*(If paying in Canadian funds,
convert using the current
exchange rate. UNESCO
coupons welcome.)*

☐ **BILL ME LATER:** ($5 service charge will be added)
(Bill-me option is good on US/Canada/Mexico orders only;
not good to jobbers, wholesalers, or subscription agencies.)

☐ Check here if billing address is different from
shipping address and attach purchase order and
billing address information.

Signature_____

☐ **PAYMENT ENCLOSED: $**_____

☐ **PLEASE CHARGE TO MY CREDIT CARD.**

☐ Visa ☐ MasterCard ☐ AmEx ☐ Discover
☐ Diner's Club

Account #_____

Exp. Date_____

Signature_____

Prices in US dollars and subject to change without notice.

NAME _____

INSTITUTION _____

ADDRESS _____

CITY _____

STATE/ZIP _____

COUNTRY _____ COUNTY (NY residents only) _____

TEL _____ FAX _____

E-MAIL_____
May we use your e-mail address for confirmations and other types of information? ☐ Yes   ☐ No

Order From Your Local Bookstore or Directly From
The Haworth Press, Inc.
10 Alice Street, Binghamton, New York 13904-1580 • USA
TELEPHONE: 1-800-HAWORTH (1-800-429-6784) / Outside US/Canada: (607) 722-5857
FAX: 1-800-895-0582 / Outside US/Canada: (607) 772-6362
E-mail: getinfo@haworthpressinc.com
PLEASE PHOTOCOPY THIS FORM FOR YOUR PERSONAL USE.